TO LOVE FASTING

TO LOVE FASTING

The Monastic Experience

Adalbert de Vogüé
Monk of La Pierre-qui-Vire

Translated from the French
AIMER LE JEÛNE, L'EXPERIENCE MONASTIQUE
by JEAN BAPTIST HASBROUCK, O.C.S.O.

CLUNY
Providence, Rhode Island

CLUNY EDITION, 2024

For more information regarding this title
or any other Cluny Media publication,
please write to info@clunymedia.com, or to
Cluny Media, P.O. Box 1664, Providence, RI 02901

ONLINE AT WWW.CLUNYMEDIA.COM

ISBN (PAPERBACK): 978-1685953522

NIHIL OBSTAT & IMPRIMI POTEST
Damase Duviller, *Abbot of La-Pierre-qui-Vire*
APRIL 1, 1986

Cover design by Clarke & Clarke
Cover image: Albrecht Dürer, *Saint Anthony Reading*,
1519, engraving
Courtesy of Wikimedia Commons

CONTENTS

To

Père Jean Gribomont, O.S.B.,

of happy and learned memory

PREFACE

THIS ESSAY is not meant to be a treatise. Putting aside the ponderous erudition with which I usually overwhelm my few readers, I describe here a personal experience, along with the meditation and research it has engendered. The learned apparatus has been reduced to the minimum. Some will find it insufficient, others still too burdensome. But I believe it is indispensable to support a reflection that does not move in the intemporal realm of ideas, but on the terrain of human history.

This essay is both precise and wide open to the infinite variety of practices that are called "fasting." Centered on one form of this, "the regular fast," it seeks to penetrate its meaning by comparison with analogous ways of behaving. In such a matter experience is everything. Therefore, I had to start with what I know from my own life. I have sought to understand this ascetical practice that has become familiar to me, the daily fast prescribed for monks by the Rule, by connecting it with its biblical and patristic origins, discussing its vicissitudes by excess or defect through the centuries, and comparing it with its non-Christian and non-religious analogues throughout the ages and in our own times.

My witness had to be personal lest I go astray by discoursing theoretically on a subject that is essentially practical. However, is not speaking of oneself not only failing in that reserve proper to Pascal's *honnête homme*, but also and especially in the secrecy that Christ recommends to his disciples? While writing I have often thought of the "hypocrites" who advertise their fasts, instead of keeping them for the Father alone to see. This evangelical advice, recalled to monks by many apophthegms, has lost none of its vigor. If I go against it, it is for the reason given, in the hope that this motive will gain me, not lose my reward.

My experience is so restrained that I scarcely expect to be praised for it. Rather, I fear that my honest description of the regular fast will make it look inferior to what it is. Perhaps I insist too much on the ease of its practice, even in our days. But this insistence at least has the advantage of dissipating a tenacious legend that today blocks the path of every attempt at the true fast, namely modern man's incapability to fast as the ancients did. If my modest witness contributes ever so little to eliminate this obstacle, I shall not regret having presented it unpretentiously. No doubt, the resulting demythologization will render the traditional practice less prestigious in the eyes of some. But if they take courage and try the experiment in their turn, it will teach them the grandeur and value of the fast better than any discourse.

I owe thanks to two young monks of my community: Brother Christopher Vuillaume, author of a master's thesis on fasting, who made useful observations on each of my chapters, and Brother Maximilian Amilon, who helped me with his medical knowledge as a physician. Besides the works cited in the footnotes, I have read with profit some articles, old and new.[1] This may serve as a bibliography in a work which, as I said before, is not scientific. On the other hand, in an appendix I give the fasting horarium of the Rule of Saint Benedict and of the Rule of the Master. This little book is not only addressed to those who live in monasteries or know the monastic life, but to every reader interested in the human and religious experience of fasting.

Perhaps some of my statements on the present state of the religious life will seem too severe. In fact, my research was born of surprise, indeed of scandal: how can the fast be totally absent from a way of life that necessarily requires it?

However, let no one see in this any opposition on principle to the modern world and to the form which monasticism has assumed in it. On the contrary, it is my place in both that demands such lucid freedom of speech. Modernity is essentially critical; therefore, to be authentically modern, we must criticize modernity.

Because of this, I feel I am performing a work of love, not of hostility. I do not aim to accuse the contemporary world and monasticism but to enrich the world with the

1. H. M. Féret, "Plaidoyer pour le jeûne," in *Prêtre et apôtre* 31 (1949), pp. 6–9; P. Miquel, "Le jeûne," in *Lettre de Ligugé* 181 (1977), p. 1–11; R. Ossart, "Le jeûne: hier et aujourd'hui," ibid., pp. 27–33.

values that monasticism can and should contribute to it. Our world needs monks who are different from itself. Please God, this essay will help them to sing more clearly and beautifully the part they have to sing in the immense symphony of the present time.

CHAPTER I

The Experience of a Solitary Monk

A day in the year of grace 1985

It is noon. As I do every day, I come down from my hermitage to the monastery, a little over half a mile away, to pick up food, books and my mail. Having risen at three o'clock, I first celebrated the night office for an hour and a half, then attended to various occupations, the heaviest of which was four hours of study. There was also Mass or communion, practical jobs, a walk and meditation, and the little hours of the Divine Office. But no breakfast: I have not eaten breakfast for almost ten years.

This noon hour provides brief contact with the community from which I have come and to which I continue to belong. Within a half hour I make the rounds of the mail box, library and kitchen, and return to my hermitage with nourishment for my mind in one arm and for my body in the other. Thus I have all I need for the next twenty-four hours. But when I return to the cell, open letters and packages, and return to study after a short siesta, the wooden container with my food in it remains closed. For six or seven years I have not eaten the noon meal.

Those afternoon hours are the best of the day. They consist of two and a half hours of intellectual work, the office of None, an hour of manual work, an hour of walking and meditating in the forest. Although fasting since the previous evening, I am at my best. One could say that the further I get from the one meal of the day, the better is my whole tone of being. My mind is at its most lucid, my body vigorous and well disposed, my heart light and full of joy. Returning from the forest about six thirty, I prepare the table and eat my meal. This consists of the four dishes my brothers had at midday: eggs or fish, vegetables, salad and fruit; I often replace one of the latter two with some cheese. I eat bread at my discretion. I eat slowly while reading, so that my meal lasts close to an hour. After that the day is almost done. All that remains is to celebrate Vespers if it is summer, to do the dishes and tidy up, to read some pages of a spiritual author and to say Compline. No matter what the season, I am in bed before nine o'clock.

The fast under discussion

The sole interest of this sketch of my horarium is the description of the fast about which I want to speak, the elementary fast that consists in eating only once a day, at the end of the day. However small it may be, this "regular fast" has been a great and joyous discovery for me, an illumination that I am happy to share.

My discovery was late, but not at all sudden. I entered the monastery at nineteen and for thirty years never omitted any of the three customary meals. The Rule of St. Benedict under which we live prescribes fasting on certain days or at certain periods, but the community imperturbably followed an horarium in which each of the three meals had its place. The calendar of the Rule, it is true, was not entirely a dead letter: when it prescribed fasting, the menu for breakfast and supper underwent some reductions, notable during Lent, rather light at other times. But this so-called "fast" was not a fast, for fasting is not eating less, but not eating at all.

The stages of discovery

It was only at the age of forty-nine, when I went from community life to solitude, that the effective fast began to enter my life. One of my desires in embracing the solitary life was to experiment with what I could do in this realm. The discrepancy between the modern observance and the prescriptions of the Rule had struck me ever since the novitiate, and no satisfactory explanation had ever been given to me. People said that man had changed; the weakness of people's health no longer allows us to fast. Was it true?

With this question in mind, I began to live alone in the spring of 1974. Timidly I began to cut down on breakfast, transferring to the other two meals what I took from it. Gradually, month by month, the first meal of the day became more and more insignificant. One day at the end of two years I suppressed the little that remained and found myself in good shape.

With this first liberation attained, I set myself to work on supper in the same way. Progressively, and in about the same length of time, I reduced it to the point where I could do without it. It was not without suspense that you make the final experiment of trying to skip a meal for the first time. One day I did without supper, and saw that all went well. Henceforth I knew that eating only once a day was possible for a modern man like me.

The next step consisted of determining the hour for the one meal. On fast days St. Benedict has the monks eat either in the middle of the afternoon ("the ninth hour," about 3 P.M.) or at the end ("evening," about 6:00 P.M.). This last time represents for him the maximum effort, what he demands in Lent, while the other constitutes a kind of attenuated fast, prescribed daily in winter and twice a week in summer. To my surprise I found out it was different for me: to fast until evening was more convenient than to eat in the middle of the afternoon. Eating a heavy meal at 3:00 P.M., as the only meal of the day has to be, means taking on a load that burdens the rest of the day. It was better to wait until evening, making the beneficial effects of the fast last as long as possible.[1]

Thus the Benedictine Lenten regime has gradually become my habitual norm, not only on the days and periods of fasting prescribed by the Rule, but every day of the

1. When a person eats shortly before going to bed, digestion accompanies sleep. The two great physiological functions are completed together, leaving the maximum of freedom to the mind during the day.

year and at every season. Indeed—and this was a new step—the advantages of all kinds that I found in fasting made me generalize this practice well beyond the limits posed by St. Benedict. Fasting was no longer a constraint and penance for me, but a joy and need of body and soul. I practiced it spontaneously because I loved it.

Sunday dinner

Thus on ordinary days I eat only once in the evening. The only exceptions are Sundays and feast days. On these days I break my fast at noon and take something in the evening, in obedience to an old Christian principle of which we shall speak later. I confess that I do this only with a sort of regret. Those days which should be the holiest, become in fact the most mediocre. In the afternoon the digestion of the meal deprives me of the incomparable lightness which characterizes the fast days. The only advantage presented by this festive horarium is to make one better disposed at the beginning of the night, and from this I profit to watch and pray a little before going to bed.

The benefits of the fast

I have alluded several times to the benefits of the fast that I practice. Now I must speak of them more explicitly. First of all, at the level of daily experience, fasting gives me singularly happy afternoons. The last phase of the twenty-four hour cycle, that immediately precedes the evening meal, is distinguished from the others by euphoria. A feeling of freedom and lightness invades my whole being, body and mind. Work, either intellectual or manual, becomes easier, as does prayer. When I walk in the forest just before the meal, while reciting the scriptural phrase that I "meditate" for that day, spiritual joy comes over me as if by appointment.

To what shall I attribute this feeling of plenitude proper to the hours of fasting? I wish I were a scientist so that I could better express it. One of my confreres sketched an explanation that attracted me: since the process of digestion is under the control of the brain, its cessation gave repose to the brain, allowed it a vacation.[2]

In fact, according to physicians, the functioning of the digestion depends less on the brain than on hormonal mechanisms and auto-regulators. However, during a fast the digestive system gets an increasing rest. About ten hours after a meal, the contractions stop and the feeling of hunger disappears; five or six hours later the glucose stops coming directly from the intestines and begins to produce itself from the reserve of glycogen contained in the liver. From then on, the body works on itself in a closed circuit, becoming itself the source of the energy it uses. Instead of destroying and appropriating to himself nourishment taken from outside,

2. Un Moine bénédictin, "Une expérience de jeûne," in *Collectanea Cisterciensia* 41 (1979), pp. 274–279 (see p. 275). Cf. my article "Aimer le jeûne. Une observance possible et nécessaire aujourd'hui," in *Collectanea Cisterciensia* 45 (1983), pp. 27–36 (see p. 33). English translation *American Benedictine Review* 35 (1984), pp. 302–313 (see p. 309).

man enters a state of nonviolence and detachment relative to the outside world.

This physiological repose, this relative isolation, this kind of autonomy and independence are singularly favorable for all activities of body and of soul. Eating three times a day means taking on, almost without respite, the work of assimilation. However light and mostly unconscious this labor of digestion is at the best of times, it nonetheless weighs continually on the psyche, and it is from this weight that fasting frees us.

Well-being and joy are therefore the most immediate effect of my daily fasts. In the long run, I also perceive a deep influence on my whole moral life.

The beneficial results of the fast are felt first in the sexual sphere. I have easily verified the connection established by the Ancients between the first two "principal vices," gluttony and lust, and consequently between the corresponding disciplines: fasting and chastity. Fasting is the most effective help for a religious who has vowed chastity. Fantasies no longer appear even during the happy hours of physiological freedom of which I have spoken, and the rest of the time they are easily controlled and eliminated.

Beyond this domain which fasting affects directly, an analogous influence is exerted over all the passions. I won't go into a detailed self-portrait, but it will surprise no one if I confess that I am subject to anxiety and irritation, sadness and nervousness, to say nothing of vanity, touchiness or envy.

The habit of fasting effects a profound appeasement of all these instinctive movements. I think the cause is that a certain mastery of the primordial appetite, eating, permits a greater mastery of the other manifestations of the libido and aggressiveness. It is as if the man who fasts were more himself, in possession of his true identity, and less dependent on exterior objects and the impulses they arouse in him.

I see now that my whole being, my physical, moral and spiritual health have benefitted by this experience of fasting, undertaken about ten years ago on the faith of the old monastic authors whom I was reading.[3] I set myself to obeying St. Benedict and the other Fathers, without knowing what awaited me. Today I know for certain that they were right.

Possible and easy today

When I consider the unfolding of my experiment, what strikes me most of all is the ease with which I have arrived at the goal. This was a surprise. At the beginning I was not even sure that I would arrive at anything that deserved to be called fasting. The word "fasting," understood in the usual and incorrect sense of which I have spoken (restrictions upon two of the three meals), reminded me painfully of the wearisome Lents when we wasted away patiently, waiting for the return of normalcy. Would the true fast that I wished to

3. Among the lesser advantages, let us note only the time saved in sitting down to table once instead of three times.

try going to resemble this wretched state, only worse? What happened was exactly the opposite. A constant, moderate, almost imperceptible effort led me to the goal without the least violence. Seldom did I labor at the task. Instead of the inconveniences and discomfort that I expected, fasting has proved to be a liberation.[4]

Thus was strikingly and unexpectedly demonstrated what I had glimpsed without being sure of it—the falseness of the current opinion that modern religious are incapable of fasting. This explanation of the actual state of contemporary religious life had always seemed suspect to me. Were we not merely salving our consciences? Was contemporary man really so weak that he lacked the physical strength to fast? I hoped to prove by experience that it is still possible to practice at least part of the abandoned observance. But I did not think it would be easy for me at the end of a short time to practice it integrally, let alone to go well beyond it.

It is now evident to me that the supposed physical weakness of modern man is a myth. If fasting is absent today from the Church and monastic life, the true cause must be sought elsewhere. Later on we shall try to get a clear view of the cause.

Fasting, when thus perceived as an expansive and liberating practice, has nothing in common with the severe

4. A slight inconvenience is the cold, to which the faster is quite sensitive, but it is nothing much. The same may be said of a certain heaviness felt upon waking when one has eaten in the evening. Although quite noticeable at the beginning, it goes away gradually.

penance it seems to be for some of my brothers. Several times people have confided to me that an attempt at fasting (whatever was meant by that) was paid for by nightmares. These violent dreams suggest that the experiment was badly carried out: the unconscious resented it as a violence. Instead of being an aggression, fasting should be felt as the suppression of useless and burdensome excess. If a person experiences its benefits, as I have, the psyche is not disturbed but strengthened and pacified.

Fasting and work

To meet other fears, perhaps I should underline that my endeavors at fasting have not caused any reduction of activity. I have never had to curtail my six or seven hours of intellectual work or renounce any physical exercise. Neither have I experienced lassitude or lessening of output at any time. It is true that I do not perform hard labor or prolonged manual work. However, a good deal of physical energy is expended in the nine miles of rapid walking I do daily, as well as in an hour of vigorous manual work, and most of this physical exertion takes place, as I have said, just during the complete fast that ends my day.

Fasting is waiting

The fast I practice therefore does not prevent work: far from it. That is because I eat what I need at my one meal. I abstain from meat, as does my community, but meat is replaced by eggs or fish. The vegetables are abundant, and my ration of bread varies between twelve and fourteen ounces. This meal with four dishes gives me quite enough calories and protein. Fasting does not mean starving oneself, but eating what is necessary at the end of a set period. Fasting is not essentially a matter of the quantity of food, but of the time when it is eaten.

Fasting and the quantity of food

Yet the quantity is also indirectly modified by fasting for it is almost impossible to eat as much in one meal as in three. However large my daily portion is, it is a notable reduction relative to the community's menu. Instead of the ten dishes that my brothers receive at their three meals, I have only five in all, including bread. This alleviation has been pure benefit for me, and it would not surprise me if it had the same effect on others.

Fasting and drinking

One point no doubt should be made clear. Every time I have spoken of fasting in Anglo-Saxon milieus where coffee and especially tea have their well-known importance, the first question asked after the conference is: "Does drinking interrupt the fast?" I have to say that the traditional fast I try to practice does exclude every liquid. The plain water that I drink with my meal suffices me for twenty-four hours. I feel no need of stimulating drinks like tea or coffee. I do without the wine that my community has on feast days, in order to have a clearer head. But these details are unimportant. The point I wish to make is that the fast as I understand it is incompatible with any drink taken outside of the one meal.[5]

The limits of an experiment

Now that I have described my experience as exactly as possible, it remains to recognize its narrow limits. The first of these pertain to my age when I began to fast: I was already forty-nine years old. The sixth decade of life, during which I made my try, is no doubt a better age than youth. In spite of the old settled habits from which more trouble could arise, one benefits from a physical and psychic maturity that makes the effort easier. The organism is more solid and stable; dietary needs tend to diminish. I do not know if I would have succeeded so easily in my twenties or even later. It is true that my weakness then may have resulted partly from an inadequate diet.

The second limit results from my solitary life. This situation, even more than age, makes things easy for me. Not only can I regulate my daily schedule and my meals as I want, but I also enjoy a calm very favorable to discipline. Passing from the common life to solitude, I found an unexpected increase

5. I count as negligible the mouthful of wine consumed at Mass early in the morning on certain days, as well as the slight host (or piece of a host when I communicate outside of Mass). For practical reasons I have not yet been able to schedule sacramental communion in the evening, just before the meal, as I would wish.

of vigor. While I was often exhausted when in community, I have almost never been since living alone, although objectively I lead a far more austere life. This observation showed me clearly the considerable amount of energy consumed by social life. To speak, to adapt to others, to be on time, to take account of one or several neighbors at every moment—all this keeps one in a state of constant, though unconscious, tension. The disappearance of these constraints frees the potential they tied up. New energies become available, and they are naturally directed towards effort exerted on oneself.

Therefore it is not hard to fast under my conditions; at least several serious obstacles were removed from my path. It is clear that this absence of common handicaps restricts my witness. In this sense I have spoken of "limits": my experience is too particular in certain ways to be easily generalized.

I must add that I enjoy good health. Without being "tough" in any sense, either physically or morally, I have the advantage of having no digestive problems and can eat a large amount of food at one time. Without this last capacity it would doubtless be impossible to sustain the regime I have described. But even accounting for all these advantages, some of which are exceptional, it seems to me that my experience of fasting is significant for my contemporaries, especially those who seek God in the Christian, religious and especially monastic life. I shall try to demonstrate this later.

The dynamics of fasting

To complete this chapter, I should note that the experiment I describe is incomplete. I describe where I am as I write. In six months, a year, two years, this stage will no doubt be surpassed.

Like any human enterprise, fasting has its natural dynamism that I have no intention of halting.

Already last year, I prolonged the fast beyond twenty-four hours. Aside from the Paschal fast (from the evening of Good Friday to Sunday morning) that causes no difficulty, I have tried six times to eat only at the end of forty-eight hours, skipping the Friday meal. The results of these weekly experiments were mixed: three times excellent, three times unpleasant. I set it aside because I do not feel ready for this kind of discipline and have sought rather to reduce my daily meal. For one Lent I easily practiced the regime prescribed by St. Benedict: two cooked and one uncooked dish. Perhaps I shall succeed in making a habit of this program of three dishes, which would reduce by one the program described above. In any case I think it healthy to keep in training by the search for the truly necessary minimum. This peaceful and constant search keeps the body healthy and the soul joyful.

Conclusion

The above is only an outline added to the description of my "regular fast," in order not to confine it within artificial boundaries. This rudimentary fast, with its present limitations, gives me sufficient matter for reflection, and I want to consider it alone in this little book. Having seen what it is, we must now locate it in the vast array of similar practices, seek its origin and meaning, trace its vicissitudes in history up to its astonishing disappearance in our era, and finally calculate its chances of restoration, and the contribution it can make to the search for God today.

CHAPTER II

The Regular Fast and Other Fasts

HAVING REPORTED my modest experience, I would like to locate it in the vast range of ancient and modern practices covered by the comprehensive term "fast." I would reproach myself for discoursing on this subject as if everything I have to say applies equally to all forms of fasting. The behavior and motives of fasters are infinitely various, and if something common unites them, their deep differences should be carefully taken into account in any honest treatment.

Therefore, I wish to begin my reflection on fasting by evoking this diversity. I do not intend to draw up a complete inventory of the different types of fasting, even if it was possible, but only to encompass a large enough view so that the specific nature of the regular fast is clear, and every equivocation removed. This preliminary clarification should allow us to sift out something useful from this one experience.

What is the regular fast?

First let us try to define the "regular fast" described in the preceding pages. The term "regular" refers to two things: (1) a rule of life and (2) the regularity of daily observance. As I said, I practiced the fast starting with the Rule of St. Benedict, clarified by its sources and by the whole context of ancient monasticism. This is a regular practice for me, since it consists in taking one meal a day at the end of the day, all year.

This definition applies to many Christian monastic observances throughout the ages. The authors of rules, beginning with St. Benedict himself, have often foreseen more flexible systems, taking into account the diversity of seasons and exempting certain times of year, particularly the exhausting days of summer. Nonetheless, the monks' fast remained regular because it was practiced continuously for long periods and because it recurred normally twice a week even in summer.

This type of habitual fast obviously implies that one meal a day is abundant enough to nourish the faster. In principle monks are obliged to work, and the fast must not prevent the six hours of manual labor or the spiritual work of the Liturgy of the Hours, called significantly "the work of God," or the work of *lectio divina*. A hallmark of the regular fast is its compatibility with all this activity. All year round, fasting and the other observances that make up the monastic life are to be practiced together.

A last trait of the regular fast is its purely religious and spiritual purpose. We shall return to fully explain this spiritual aspect later. But from the start we must take note of a motive that differs visibly from those to which we are accustomed by the most frequent kinds of fasts of our days, whether they be medical fasts or those of political protest.

Let us now see how the principal experiences of fasting that have arisen in the three to four thousand years of the Judeo-Christian tradition compare with this "regular fast."

Fasting in the Bible

Nothing could be more different than the models of fasting in the Bible. Most often, Biblical fasts are transient and only for a single day, occasioned by a fortuitous, determinate event.

Yom Kippur

The only regular fast prescribed by the Mosaic Law is that of the Day of Atonement (Yom Kippur), the tenth day of the seventh month, usually September on our modern calendar.[1] It is celebrated once a year and is limited to that one day. In this case as well as in most of those about which we shall speak, it consists simply in eating nothing until evening for one day, and is accompanied by the prohibition of work.

Occasional fasts

Fasts in the Bible are sometimes occasioned by mourning[2] or by an anguished situation in which one wishes

1. Nm 29:7; Lv 16:29–31; 23:27–30. Cf. Acts 27:9.
2. 2 Sm 1:12 (death of Saul and Jonathan); 2 Sm 3:35 (death of Abner). Cf. 2 Sm 12:16–23, where David's entourage wrongly counts on the king fasting after the death of his child.

to obtain the maximum intensity and efficacy for prayer. When a fault has been committed or heaven's punishment incurred,[3] on the eve of battle or following a defeat,[4] in preparation for a long and dangerous journey, or when faced with the death of a loved one,[5] every dramatic circumstance calls for supplication reinforced by fasting. To fasting is often added, as in mourning, weeping, rending garments, wearing haircloth, sleeping on sackcloth, putting ashes on one's head, and abstaining from bathing and the use of oil.[6] All of these, but especially fasting, "humbles the soul," giving convincing proofs of distress and devotion to touch God's heart.

This fast, accompanied by prayer, can be done by an individual or a community. In the second case, a decree is issued that obliges each member: "a fast is proclaimed" so that all may observe it.[7] If the duration is not mentioned, we can assume it is "until evening," a phrase that appears here and there,[8] confirming that it is a single day's fast.

---

3. 1 Kgs 21:27–29 (Ahab); Jon 3:5–7; Cf. 1 Kgs 21:9,12; Jl 1:14 and 2:15.
4. 1 Sm 7:6; 1 Mc 3:47; Jgs 20:26. See also 1 Sm 14:24.
5. Ezr 8:21–23; 2 Sm 12:16–22.
6. 1 Kgs 21:27–29; 1 Mc 3:47.
7. 1 Kgs 21:9,12; 2 Chr 20:3; Jon 3:5; Is 58:5; Jer 36:9; Ezr 8:21. Cf. Jl 1:14 and 2:15 ("to sanctify a fast").
8. Jgs 20:26; 2 Sm 1:12 and 3:35 (cf. 1 Sm 14:24). See also Is 58:5 ("one fast" = "one day").

Commemorations

Alongside these one-day practices tied to the unforeseeable vicissitudes of life, there appear after the Exile some commemorative fasts in the yearly calendar like that of Yom Kippur. In the fourth month the breach of the walls of Jerusalem in 587 is celebrated; in the fifth month the capture of the city; in the seventh the assassination of Gedaliah; in the tenth the beginning of the siege.[9] These commemorations of those two terrible years, recurring on fixed dates, engender a rough outline of the regular fast: although they are one-day events, the practice already has the character of an observance. It is the same for fast commemorating the salvation of the nation obtained by Esther, but this fast of the month Adar (February–March) does not affect only one day, but two days in a row (Est 9:31).

When the regular fast commemorates the national catastrophe of the sixth century, it assumes an aspect of mourning which reminds us of the funeral rites mentioned above. This fast, motivated by an irreparable misfortune, does not have the same meaning as the fast which sustains an urgent prayer. Fasting because one has lost a close relative without hope of recalling him, is simply to show that a great sorrow has cut off one's appetite, taken away the taste for living and eating, suspended the most fundamental acts of life. Although physiological in origin, the refusal of food in such

9. Zec 7:5 and 8:19.

a case can of course become a simple gesture of decorum. Ranging from an incapacity to eat because of the emotion choking one's throat, to a mere conformity to custom, fasting because of a death can be more or less detached from its organic substratum and become more or less a convention.

Fasting for more than one day: prolongations and repetitions

For one who has in mind the monks' regular fast, it is particularly interesting to pick out among these many examples of one-day fasts some cases where the act is prolonged or repeated beyond one day. The Book of Esther, in which we have already met with two successive days of fasting serving as an annual commemoration, reports that Esther's decisive intervention with the king was preceded by three days of continual fasting, observed not only by the queen but also, at her orders, by all the Jews in the capital (Est 4:16). This time it was not a juxtaposition of several days of distinct fasts (which I call "repetition"), but "not eating or drinking for three days and three nights" (which I call "prolongation"). Similarly during the seven-day sickness of his infant son, David seems to have refused all nourishment (2 Sm 12:16–23). In other passages there are also fasts of "three days" or of "seven," but each of these days could have ended with a meal.[10]

10. 2 Mc 13:12; 1 Sm 7:6 and 1 Chr 10:12.

These two types of fasting, prolonged or repeated, are also found on a greater scale in certain pages of the Bible. The "forty days" of Moses and of Jesus are explicitly of the first type,[11] while the "many days" of Nehemiah and the "three weeks" of Daniel belong no doubt to the second,[12] which is closer to the "regular fast."

The first regular fasts

However, all these periods of fasting have an episodic character which contrasts them with our observance. The latter is truly outlined in a very small number of texts, which are the more remarkable for being so rare. First, there is Judith's fast which accompanied her widowhood, which has lasted three years and four months when she enters the scene in the Biblical narrative: "She fasted every day, except for the sabbaths, new moons and the feasts of the house of Israel." At the beginning of the New Testament another widow does the same, even to extreme old age: "night and day Anna served the Lord in fasts and prayers."[13]

Besides these apparently daily fasts, St. Luke's Gospel mentions the "twice a week fasts" about which the Pharisee boasted (Lk 18:12). This fast is less frequent, but not less regular. These regular fasts contrast with the occasional practices

11. Ex 34:28 (cf. 24:18); Dt 9:9 and 18; Mt 4:2; Lk 4:12; See also 1 Kgs 19:8 (Elijah).

12. Neh 1:4; Dn 10:2–3 (simple abstinence from wine and meat?).

13. Jdt 8:6; Lk 2:37.

mentioned by the same Luke both among the Christians and their enemies, whether it be fasts (of one day?) preceding an assignment to missionary work, a departure for the missions, a separation, or a kind of fast until death vowed by the forty fanatics of Jerusalem who wish to assassinate Paul.[14]

Different aspects of the fast

In closing this Scriptural panorama of fasting I must note that in the Bible fasting often has a very different physiognomy than the one described in the preceding chapter according to my experience. It is an exceptional act, provoked by extraordinary circumstances—usually it is linked with misfortune. Far from being a happy and expansive experience, it appears as a way of "humbling (or afflicting) one's soul," accompanied by tears and other expressions of sorrow. People fast when disaster draws near, to obtain its removal; and when it has already happened, to weep over it (mourning) or to avoid its aggravation or repetition. Because of its unusual character, fasting entails fatigue or weakness: warriors are hampered or even prevented from fighting.[15] It is accompanied by the interruption of normal activities: the single fast prescribed by the Law takes place on a day without work, when the sabbath rest is imposed.

14. Acts 13:2–3 and 14:23; 23:12.
15. 1 Sm 14:24–30; 1 Mc 3:17.

This usual aspect of fasting in the Bible, which contrasts so strongly with what I have known of it, still does not exclude other aspects in which I find more of my point of view. The fast of Judith and Anna is not only "regular," as mine is, but it is linked to celibacy and prayer in a way that is already very monastic. The solitary fasts of Moses on the mountain, and of Elijah and of Jesus in the desert also speak to a monk's heart, inasmuch as the first two are a prelude to a meeting with God, and the third, which follows the theophany of the baptism in the Jordan, takes place under the motion of the Holy Spirit. Even though Daniel's fasts are accompanied by lamentations, they also precede revelations, and it is probably for the same purpose, to dispose oneself to receive a message from on high, that the prophets in Antioch fast before letting Saul and Barnabas depart.

In the Early Days of Christianity

Before passing from the New Testament to the Christian Church, there is one author, contemporary with Christ, who deserves to be listened to very carefully, Philo the Jew. According to him,[16] the *Therapeutae* of Alexandria, genuine monks before their time, already observed a truly regular fast

16. Philo, *De vita contemplativa*, 34–37 (cf. 64–71; 81–82).

which coincides almost exactly with the observance I have described, while surpassing it in more than one respect.

The Therapeutae *of Philo*

These *Therapeutae* were Jewish ascetics, men and women, forming a sort of semi-eremitic colony in lower Egypt; they ate every day only after sunset, "for they judge philosophy to be worthy of the light and bodily needs worthy of darkness." Since we know that the twice-a-week fast of Judaism, like the occasional Jewish fasts about which we have just spoken, consisted of eating nothing before evening, it seems that this daily evening meal of the *Therapeutae*, aside from its "philosophical" motive, is the generalization of a contemporary Jewish custom. What the Pharisee of the Gospel did twice a week, these monks did every day.

However, certain *Therapeutae* went further. Their "love of learning" pushed them to eat only every three days, and some even "found so much delight in feasting on wisdom" that they doubled this time and took food only at the end of six days. These prolonged fasts were more remarkable in that the menu was extremely austere. For everyone it was bread and salt with water to drink; the more delicate added only an herb, the hyssop plant.

Under all these aspects this regime is of the greatest interest to one seeking to understand the practices of Christian monasticism, for we shall see that Philo's narrative, inserted two centuries later into Eusebius' *Ecclesiastical History*, inspired, if not the experiences of the first monks, at least the literary image given to them in works destined to exert an immense influence, such as those of Athanasius and Cassian. For the present let us be content to note the diverse modes of the fast in honor with these Jewish precursors: to the one meal of the day taken in the evening is added the diet of bread and water, while this already rigorous observance is stiffened by days and almost weeks of absolute fasting among the more fervent.

The contemplative aspiration which motivates this enthusiastic discipline is not to be neglected either. For all its being formulated in Greek terms such as "philosophy, love of learning, the delights of wisdom," its concrete support is nonetheless the reading and interpretation of the Bible, practiced all day long by each *Therapeutae* in his own "monastery." We think of the word of Deuteronomy repeated by Jesus when fasting in the desert: "One does not live by bread alone but by every word that comes from the mouth of God."[17] The Christian monks of Egypt in their turn will spend their days repeating passages of Scripture learned by heart, nourishing their soul with the divine word while their stomach remains fasting. Thus for this whole tradition, fasting has in scriptural "meditation" its necessary accompaniment to help and direct its effort.

17. Dt 8:3; Mt 4:4.

The Didache *and Tertullian: the "stations"*

Another witness, a little later than Philo's, is almost as important for the history of the Christian fast, that of the *Didache*. In this little writing of the apostolic age, fasting is prescribed not only for one or two days before baptism, but twice a week as in Judaism. Instead of fasting on Monday and Thursday as do "the hypocrites," meaning the Jews, Christians will fast on Wednesdays and Fridays.[18] That is the first attestation of a practice that will structure the week for the entire ancient church as well as for monasticism.

It seems quite evident that this witness should be related to the evangelical text already mentioned, the prayer of the Pharisee in which he congratulates himself on fasting twice a week. These two fast days were not specified by St. Luke, but we learn here that they were Mondays and Thursdays. Christianity has therefore both made this Jewish observance its own, and modified it. The two days substituted for those of Judaism are obviously chosen for their relation to Christ's passion. The relation is obvious in regard to Friday, but it is equally affirmed with regard to Wednesday, with some variations of detail, either the betrayal by Judas or the arrest of Jesus. The first Christians thus realized the Lord's prediction: "The days will come, when the bridegroom will

18. *Didache* 7:4 (pre-baptismal fast, cf. Justin, *Apol.* 1,61; Clement, *Recogn.* III, 67, 3); 8, 1 (weekly fast). See also 1, 3 (paraphrase of Mt 5:44); 6:3 (permitted and forbidden foods).

be taken away from them, and then they will fast in those days."[19]

Yet this twice-weekly fast differed from that of the Jews in other ways. The most important difference is the new time assigned to the meal that ends it: instead of waiting until evening as the Jews did, Christians ate from the ninth hour onward, in the middle of the afternoon. The Christian fast of Wednesdays and Fridays was therefore only a "semi-fast," as it was sometimes called.

The motive of this attenuation was less a desire for ease, it seems, than a care to preserve the secret character of the fast, as the Lord had taught.[20] Fasting was a free observance and to be meritorious, it should not be publicized. But the *cena* or evening meal, which was the principal meal of the day, was eaten from the ninth hour onward. One could therefore, without being much noticed, omit the two secondary meals preceding it, which were more or less optional, the *ientaculum* or breakfast, and the *prandium* or midday meal, and eat with everyone else from the ninth hour on, thus concealing one's renunciation from the eyes of men.

These modalities of the twice-a-week fast, called "the station," are well known to us by means of the little treatise in which Tertullian, already a Montanist, criticizes them

19. This plural (Lk 5:35) is read in certain witnesses of Mk 2:20, whose primitive text seems to be in the singular ("that day").

20. Mt 6:16–18. On the following, see J. Schummer, *Die altchristliche Fastenpraxis* (Münster, 1933), LQF 27, p. 102–104.

severely.[21] In the worldwide church from which he had separated himself, the stational fast was optional and did not go beyond the ninth hour. A little earlier, around 200, when Tertullian was still a Catholic priest, he had pointed out and discussed in his treatise *On Prayer* another particularity of this observance: the Christians who fasted abstained from the Eucharistic celebration in order to avoid breaking their fast by receiving Communion.[22] Tertullian advised against this abstention and offered them a means to reconcile everything: by reserving the consecrated species received at Mass to consume them only at the ninth hour, they could observe their fast without depriving themselves of the Eucharistic celebration and Communion.

Lent, Vigils, Ember Days, Rogation Days

To this habit of fasting twice a week, which goes back to the very origins of the Church, were joined other practices which we need not describe in detail since they are familiar to us. I am thinking in particular of the celebration of Lent and Ember Days which have continued down to our own times.

Lent originated in the complete fast of one or two days preceding the feast of Easter. It was extended first to one week, then to three, and ended by comprising forty days, in memory of Christ's forty days in the wilderness. And

21. Tertullian, *De ieiunio.*

22. Tertullian, *De oratione* 19.

since baptism was administered during the night of the Paschal vigil, this fast in preparation for Easter served also as a pre-baptismal fast. As we have seen, the *Didache* already prescribed fasting for one or two days before baptism, inviting all the faithful to associate themselves, as far as they could, with the preparatory fast of their future brothers.

Even when the Lenten fast was later imposed on the whole church, the Paschal fast proper, that is, the whole of Holy Saturday until the vigil service,[23] retained its special character of rigorous obligation. At the end of the sixth century, poor St. Gregory, who felt too ill to observe it, experienced an unspeakable shame at the thought that even the little children remained fasting on that day.[24]

This supremely sacred observance, the Paschal fast, refers to the words of Jesus already mentioned: "The days will come when the bridegroom is taken away from them, and then they will fast in those days." On the eve of baptism we might also think of another word from the Gospel: "This kind of devil can come out only through prayer and fasting."[25] Baptism as renunciation of Satan calls for this kind of exorcism which fasting is, and this remark can apply beyond Holy Saturday to the whole pre-baptismal period of Lent.

23. Cf. Cassian, *Conferences* 21, 25,3.

24. Gregory the Great, *Dialogues* III, 33,7.

25. Mt 17:21. "Fasting" is absent in the parallel place in Mk 9:29.

When new feasts, ranged throughout the year, were added to the unique feast of Easter, the more important ones were given days of anticipation, improperly called vigils, and the fasts observed on them imitated the Paschal fast. The fast of the Ember Days, which St. Leo in the middle of the fifth century thought should be attributed to the apostles, were in reality, like Lent, a relatively late institution, incorporating a very ancient element. This latter element was none other than the stational fast of Wednesday and Friday, to which a specifically Roman custom added Saturday. The aim of these celebrations, which occurred every three months, was to solemnize the four seasons of the year, to which was added the memory of the biblical fast of the fourth, seventh and tenth months. But whatever the motives given for each of these four Ember weeks and for the whole group of them, they were chiefly a recall of the ancient and venerable "stations" of each week, surviving at long intervals in a Christian world which was abandoning them.

The fasts of the Ember seasons, like the stational fast, were accompanied by common prayer, according to the biblical tradition so well summed up by Jesus' words, "prayer and fasting." The union of these two sacred acts was so natural and necessary that one of them could scarcely be practiced without the other. This is quite evident in the case of the rogation days. Originally they were merely days of prolonged prayer. People interrupted the prayer to eat, and the meal lowered the spiritual tension and made the prayer mediocre. In the third quarter of the fifth century, a bishop of Vienne in Gaul, St. Mamertus, remedied this trouble by suppressing the dinner. The rogation prayers, thus associated with fasting, immediately assumed a remarkable dignity and efficacy. Although Sidonius Apollinaris was little given to asceticism personally, he could not help but congratulate the bishop of Vienne and introduce into his own church of Clermont these liturgies of supplication renewed by fasting.[26]

The First Monks

We must add the special fasts of the monks to these customs which in principle concern the whole Christian people. Without entering into the history of the regular fast, which we shall consider later, let us at least point out some facts that give an idea of the context in which this type of fast developed.

Anthony and Palamon

Like the *Therapeutae* of Philo, St. Anthony, the first Christian hermit whose life was recounted, was not content to observe the minimal rule of one meal a day in the evening. From the beginning of his ascetic life, St. Athanasius shows him fasting, sometimes two or even four days in a row. Whether his

26. Sidonius Apollinaris, *Letters* 5, 14, 2–3; 7, 1, 2 (written in 473).

meals were daily or less often, they consisted of only bread, salt and water.

In the same way, St. Pachomius, who was to become the father of the cenobites, began the monastic life with an old anchorite named Palamon, whose rule for fasting was to eat every day in summer, but only every other day in winter, and he would not stand for adding a single drop of oil to the salt, even on Easter Sunday.[27]

Jerusalem in the time of Egeria

Towards the end of the fourth century, the regime of many *apotactites* (ascetics) in Jerusalem, both men and women, was no less rigorous, at least in Lent. According to the traveler Egeria, those who fasted all week (the *hebdomadaries*) formed a separate group, numerous enough to have the time of the public Mass on Saturday advanced out of regard for them. Only after this dawn Mass did they break their fast which had lasted since the dinner of the preceding Sunday.

At these two meals for the week, the early meal on Saturday and the noon meal on Sunday, these great Lenten fasters took only water and a little porridge made of flour. The same severe abstinence was observed by those who ate

27. Athanasius, *Life of Anthony* 7, 6; *First Greek Life of St. Pachomius* (G^1) 6–7, Cistercian Studies 45 (Kalamazoo, MI: Cistercian Publications, 1980), pp. 301–302.

28. Egeria, *The Pilgrimage of Egeria*, 27, 9–28, 4.

more often, adding to the two meals mentioned a supper on Thursday, or sometimes Wednesday or even every evening.[28]

The regimes of Hilarion and others

Unfortunately, these Lenten regimes are the only ones reported by Egeria. We must turn to other documents to learn how monks and nuns lived the rest of the year. There are many of them, for there is scarcely any Life of the saints which does not speak, sometimes very precisely, about the hero's eating habits.

It even happens that his successive regimes are set before our eyes in a list. Thus Jerome, towards the beginning of the Life of Hilarion, divides the long life of the holy man into five periods, and for each of them he shows the daily menu. The longest period, from age thirty-four to sixty-two, comprised "six ounces of barley bread and one green vegetable lightly cooked in oil, without any fruit or dry vegetable or anything else whatsoever."[29] Of course there was only one meal a day, but Hilarion distinguished himself by never eating it before sunset, not even on feast days or in his gravest sicknesses.

The two great collections of monastic historiography of the fourth and fifth centuries, the *Historia Monachorum in Aegypto*[30] and the *Lausiac History* also describe a goodly

29. Jerome, *Life of Hilarion* 5, 4. Six ounces make a Roman half-pound, or about one hundred and sixty-five grams, or 5.82 oz. avoirdupois.

30. English translation, *The Lives of the Desert Fathers*, Cistercian Studies 34 (Kalamazoo, MI: Cistercian Studies, 1981).

number of various regimes. The most frequent trait, which comes up in almost every mention, is *omophagia*, or the refusal of all cooked food except bread, and sometimes even without excepting that. Another famous report on Egyptian monasticism, John Cassian's, speaks of a norm quite generally observed by the hermits, having been recognized by experience as the best. Every day the hermit takes a pound of bread (a little more than three hundred and twenty grams (11.3 ounces)), half at the ninth hour and half in the evening. No other food is added to this dry bread, which is considered as the surest guarantee of faultless chastity. If the hermit takes the ration in two stages, contrary to the rule of only one meal, it is for particular reasons of hospitality which Cassian explains. The latter notes also that in this way one feels lighter in celebrating the evening and night offices.[31]

All these ascetical programs, as we see, combine fasting properly so-called, which pertains to the hour of the meal, with abstinences which are sometimes very rigorous and a rationing of quantity that can be Draconian. Under these conditions we are not surprised to learn that the first great Egyptian monk described in the *Historia*, the famous prophet recluse John of Lyco, was extremely thin, and almost hairless and beardless. The "pallor" caused by fasting is a usual trait in the monks' portraits, and St. Basil, who notes it among his own monks, also emphasizes their

31. Cassian, *Conferences* 2, 19–26.

physical weakness; thus the labor expected of well-fed men cannot be demanded of them.[32]

This last trait is a little suspect, for it appears in a request for a reduction of taxes, but it is evident that the dietary restrictions of every kind included in the fast tended to make it, even in a moderate cenobitic milieu like Basil's, a cause of permanent weakness. Again this is a trait I must point out the more carefully, since it is far from my own experience.

Melania the Younger and the Monks of Palestine

To complete this survey of the monastic world of the first centuries, it will suffice to point out some of the peaks which stand out among many others. From the time of her conversion to asceticism, the great Roman lady Melania the Younger took upon herself stricter and stricter fasts, at first eating only once a day in the evening, then every other day, and finally every five days, that is, Saturdays and Sundays. Thus she successively made her own the different renunciations that Egeria, thirty years earlier, saw practiced by the ascetics of Jerusalem during Lent. To mark Lent, Melania added to the week-long fast the use of barley bread and abstinence from oil.[33]

In the same way St. Euthymius, the great founder of Palestinian monasteries in the fifth century, habitually ate

32. Basil, *Long Rules* 17, 2; *Letters* 46, 2 and 284.

33. Gerontius, *Life of Melania* 22 and 24. That was in Africa, about 410.

nothing five days out of seven. His disciple, St. Sabas, did the same from the age of thirty onward, during the five years (469–474) when he led the solitary life in a grotto, close to the community which had formed him. His fast was accompanied by work, for each week he made fifty baskets. When he became the superior of a *laura*, he took up the habit of wandering in the desert all during Lent, and nourished himself during this time only with Communion on Saturdays and Sundays.

One of his monks, the famous John the Hesychast, also passed the week without any meals except on Saturday and Sunday. This regime is attested to during the three years (493–495) when he lived as a solitary near Sabas, but it seems also to have been his rule for other periods, notably during some fifty years of seclusion, beginning in 509, at the end of his life. Indeed, he was over a hundred years old when he died.[34]

Longevity indeed is an habitual fact among these great Palestinian monks for whom Cyril of Scythopolis has furnished us with a very sure and precise chronology. Euthymius lived to ninety-six, Sabas to ninety-three, and both of them accomplished considerable labors as founders and superiors. This is a sign that extreme austerity does not prevent good health or even the unfolding of a fruitful activity.

34. Cyril of Scythopolis, *Life of Euthymius* 21; *Life of Sabas* 10 and 24; *Life of John the Hesychast* 7 and 28. Cistercian Studies 114 (Kalamazoo, MI: Cistercian Publications, 1991).

It is true that Euthymius and Sabas, like all the heroes of Cyril of Scythopolis, lived and worked habitually in the semi-eremitic framework of the *laura*, where silence and solitude enveloped the five working days of the week. Their astonishing vitality is inseparable from these conditions.

The Lents of Simeon Stylites

At the time of Euthymius and in the neighboring country of Syria, one last peak irresistibly draws our attention: the performances of Simeon the Stylite, whose renown was immense. Before and after he mounted his famous pillar, people saw him pass entire Lents without eating anything, after the example of Jesus.

The progression of these heroic attempts is significant. At the end of his first Lent, Simeon was found lying unconscious, flat on the floor of his cell near the food he had not wished to touch. Later, year by year, little by little, he mastered the total fast, succeeding at first in remaining conscious, then in remaining standing and in prayer. To achieve that, he began by tying himself and thus keeping himself erect; later he achieved the same results by his own strength.[35] It was a magnificent conquest of self, which confirms that in this domain, as in many others, everything, or almost everything, is a matter of habit.

35. Theodoret, *History of the Monks of Syria*. Cistercian Studies 88 (Kalamazoo, MI: Cistercian Publications, 1985), pp. 163–164.

This extreme case plainly shows the fatigue and suffering that can accompany fasting. In such a case we are far from the euphoric little exercise described in the preceding chapter. It is good to look squarely into the suffering face of the fast. Even in the cenobitic milieu its afflictive aspect often appears, whether it is used as a punishment for faults, or to sustain, as in the Bible, an insistent supplication in time of distress.[36]

Fasting in the Twentieth Century

Let us complete this survey by a glance at our own times. While the traditional practice of fasting in the Catholic Church has completed its self-degradation and has ended in quasi-suppression, other milieux have preserved or even developed diverse forms of fasting.

The Laws of the Church

Before World War II, one could still see Christians observing the rules of the ecclesiastical fast conscientiously, although apparently without enthusiasm. Lent, the Ember days and vigils were announced from the pulpit, and the faithful who did not enjoy one of the numerous exemptions—too young,

36. *The Rule of the Master*, Cistercian Studies 6 (Kalamazoo, MI: Cistercian Publications, 1977), 13, 50–53, etc. (punishment); 15, 39–47 (supplication).

too old, insufficient health, a job that was reckoned as hard labor—rationed their breakfast and their supper, reducing the latter to a simple "collation," as they said.

Was this fasting? Certainly not, properly speaking, if the fast signifies absence of nourishment. Although resented by many as a painful privation, the Church fast could be very meritorious, but it was not a fast. After centuries of accommodations which had ruined the fundamental principle of one meal a day, ecclesiastical law no longer obtained for those who observed it the experience and benefit of a true fast.

A Eucharistic fast also existed, and it had its uses. To have abstained from food and drink since midnight was the condition of being able to receive Communion. This effort to remain fasting, whether great or small according to the time when Mass was celebrated, represented in any case a homage paid to the Sacrament, a sign of the value attached to it, a reminder of its incomparable dignity.

But the rule had troublesome effects on participation in the Eucharist and on the time of the celebrations. Reception of Communion usually did not prevail when placed in the balance with breakfast, and only the Masses celebrated early could count on a reasonable number of communicants. Moreover, since the Eucharist was never celebrated in the afternoon at that time, the Eucharistic fast was a sort of semi-fast, as the ancients used to say.

Ramadan

Although the true fast is practically absent from Catholic life these days, it has survived and continues to survive in the Moslem world. The twenty-nine or thirty days of Ramadan when people eat nothing before sunset, constitute a social and spiritual fact of great importance.

Yet observations dating from more than a quarter of a century ago, which no doubt would be corroborated by recent inquiries, show a conflict between religious law and the modern world.[37] The fast of Ramadan is thought fatiguing, and is said to be ill-suited to habitual work, which has to be reduced or slowed.

This remark should be compared with what I said in the first chapter. In itself the Ramadan fast is not more fatiguing than my "regular fast," since the Koran does not forbid eating one's fill once night has come. The possibility of eating at the end of the night as well as at the beginning even makes this observance much less burdensome than mine. But not being used to it no doubt explains that people find it difficult to maintain a normal rhythm of work as I do constantly and without trouble. It is one thing to fast one month a year, and another to do it every day.

37. J. Jomier and J. Corbon, *Le Ramadan au Caire en 1956* (extracts reproduced by P. R. Régamey, *Redécouverte du jeûne* [Paris, 1959], pp. 337–342). See also G. Farès, "Le jeûne de ramadan," in *Lettre de Ligugé* 18 (January 1977), p. 12–26.

Hinduism and Gandhi

Another great religion, Hinduism, keeps alive the tradition of fasting. At the beginning of his *Experiences of Truth*, Gandhi evokes some of the familiar practices of his native land, such as the fast of *ekadashi* (the eleventh day of the fifteen-day lunar cycle) or the devotional fasts of his mother, which were sometimes heroic.[38]

But Gandhi's *Autobiography* interests us, especially in what it tells of his own undertakings in this field. Not only does the work abound with notes about diet, but it reports the first attempts at the prolonged fasts of this man who was to make such spectacular ones.

It is significant that the first two fasts of a social character by Gandhi were fasts of penitence: first one week (1913), and then two (1914), to make reparation for the grave faults committed by the young people for whom he felt responsible. This penitential motive remained dominant in the series of his later fasts, of which there were a half-dozen of the same type. He noted that the week in 1913 effected the purification of the atmosphere around him as well as pacifying him interiorly. Moreover he did not halt his activity, and to these seven days of complete fast added the vow to take only one meal a day for four and a half months, while strictly maintaining his diet, which comprised only fruit. The two weeks

38. Mohandas K. Gandhi, *An Autobiography: The Story of My Experiments with Truth* (Boston, MA: Beacon Press, 1957), pp. 4–5 (Part I, Ch. 1) and 33 (I, Ch. 10). (Cf. 320 [IV, Ch. 27,3] and 330 [IV, Ch. 31, 3].)

in 1914 ended more painfully: he could only talk in a very low voice and had recourse to dictation instead of writing.[39]

These first episodes, which took place in South Africa, already show several traits that are constantly found in Gandhi's fasts: their public character combined with deep interior motives; extreme delicacy of conscience, combining inflexible principles with the most subtle considerations and nuances; the context of precarious health and very austere abstinence that made these extraordinary fasts a gamble, a genuine risk, since the man undertaking them was frail and recovered afterwards only with difficulty.

Gandhi's first two fasts after his return to India were no less significant. They were both for only three days, but they differed in occasion and in nature. While the second one in April 1919, to make reparation for acts of popular violence, extended the domestic penances of the African period to Indian political life, the first one (March 1918) aimed at helping the strikers who were beginning to lose heart.[40]

In undertaking the latter, Gandhi set no term for himself: he would not stop until a settlement was reached or the strikers left the mills. Apparently there was pressure involved, but the impact on the mill-owners, who happened to be Gandhi's friends, was not willed for itself or even held

39. Ibid., pp. 342–344 (IV, Ch. 36 entire).

40. Ibid., pp. 426–434, March 1918 (V, Ch. 20–22); p. 468, April 1919 (V, 32, fifth paragraph before end).

to be legitimate. It was "the grave defect" of this fast that it exerted such pressure, because of the circumstances, and this pressure was a form of violence. Gandhi's intention was simply to bear in his own flesh the moral failure of the strikers who were failing in their pledge not to return to work before having obtained satisfaction.

This action remained basically, in spite of appearances, in the penitential line of the practices already described. However, its spectacular result—the reconciliation of the two parties after three days—revealed the fearful moral power of the unlimited fast, practiced on this occasion for the first time. By its mode and its results, the experiment foretells the fasts until death of 1932 and 1948.

Before and after his triduum of 1919, Gandhi called for collective fasts of twenty-four hours, on a national or local scale, for the sake of purification or penitence.[41] "The Muslims may not fast for more than one day," he noted the first time, "therefore we must set this limit on the fast." Moreover, never did he request anyone to fast for more than one day,[42] although his own periods of fasting several times lasted as long as three weeks (1921, 1933, 1943).

41. Ibid., pp. 459–460 (V, Ch. 30, third paragraph before end); p. 468 (V, Ch. 32, fifth paragraph before end).

42. C. Drevet, "Les jeûnes de Mahatma Gandhi" in Régamey, *Redécouverte,* pp. 249–296 (see p. 282). To this general survey can be added the list of Gandhi's fasts in the introduction to M. K. Gandhi, *Expériences de vérité ou Autobiographie,* trad. G. Belmont (Paris, 1950). (This list of fasts does not exist in the English translation mentioned in n. 41.)

We would love to continue following this prodigious personality in his experiments and reflections on the matter. Let us at least note the essential role of personal motives of a spiritual character in his practice of ordinary fasting and abstinence. The medical preoccupations, which were at first predominant or even exclusive, were soon replaced by higher cares, tied to the ideal and vow of chastity, This vow, pronounced in 1906 at the age of thirty-seven, was at the heart of a search for total purity, demanding a limitless interior effort, which recognized that it was dependent on the grace of God.

Gandhi has spoken better than anyone of both the necessity and insufficiency of the physical fast.[43] But the same can be said of many other aspects of the problem of food in its relation to the life of the soul. The life and works of Gandhi are so rich in this regard that they can be considered a microcosm collecting almost everything useful that has been experienced and said on the question throughout the ages.

Religion and therapy

To complete this summary overview, it suffices to mention two forms of fasting which are alive in the contemporary West: the therapeutic fast and the political fast.

43. Gandhi, *Autobiography*, pp. 209–211 (III, Ch. 8, paragraph 5 to the end); pp. 325–332 (IV, Ch. 29–31 entire).

Specifically religious fasting has not completely disappeared. The recent apparitions of the Virgin at Medjugorje have even restored to honor the ancient observance of fasting on bread and water on Wednesday and Friday. But western Christianity remains deprived of living customs and spiritual motives, and Christians interested in fasting are usually reduced to searching for an inspiration in the past or taking one of the secular ways of which we are going to speak.

The medical practice is based on the healing effect of "autodigestion" entailed in fasting. As Alexis Carrel already wrote, fasting "purifies and profoundly modifies our tissues."[44] The doctors who use this method are not afraid of prolonged fasts, but some hold that a brief and frequent fast is more helpful.[45]

When reading the medical literature on the subject, it sometimes seems that the regular fast of the monastic tradition is excluded by the very definition given of the fast. If, as one doctor writes, "the fast is the interruption of the normal rhythm of meals,"[46] to fast every day, that is, to make fasting the normal rhythm of one's meals, seems like a contradiction

44. A. Carrel, *L'Homme, cet inconnu* (Paris, 1935), p. 274. English translation, *Man the Unknown*, Ch. VI, section 12, MacFadden edition (1961), p. 151.

45. Cf. T. Ryan, *Fasting Rediscovered: A Guide to Health and Wholeness for Your Body-Spirit* (New York, 1982), pp. 97–99: one day a week would be best.

46. J. Trémolières, "Aspects physiologiques du jeûne," in Régamey, *Redécouverte*, pp. 195–210 (see p. 195).

in terms. In the monastic milieu it would be necessary then to reserve the name of "fast" to some exceptional practices, for example, the increase of austerity during Lent.

Although Carrel did not formulate for himself this reductive definition, he seems to have something analogous in mind when he praises the benefits of meals "sometimes abundant, sometimes scanty."[47] The rather rarified monastic regimes of which I spoke above, do not follow this principle of variation. Regularity in eating is even vigorously inculcated by many an ancient author, and by Cassian in particular.

We shall have to take into account this conception of the fast and its advantages when we later reflect on the traditional way of fasting in monasticism. For now it suffices to observe that the "normal" rhythm, that is, the usual rhythm of contemporary man consists in eating three times a day.[48] Relative to that, the one daily meal of the regular fast does indeed represent "an interruption." Such a rupture is still effective even if it is permanent. Perhaps the regular fast is not one if we consider the present habits of the faster, but it is very real if we refer to the general custom of his contemporaries, which was once that of the faster himself.

47. A. Carrel, *L'Homme, cet inconnu*, p. 276. English translation, p. 151. Same praise of variation in the anonymous study "Expérience et réflexions postérieures d'un religieux prisonnier de guerre," in Régamey, *Redécouverte*, pp. 349–379 (see pp. 361–362).

48. An equivalence which stands out clearly in J. Trémolières, "Aspects physiologiques du jeûne," p. 195, for whom this "normality" is only a matter of fact (he underlines the artificial nature of our law of three meals a day).

The Political Fast

Following Gandhi, fasting has become an instrument of political protest and pressure. There is no need to expound on a phenomenon that is sufficiently widespread to catch everyone's attention. Let us only note that this practice, which is so alive at present, is itself very diverse. Not only do we distinguish here, as in Gandhi's life, simple public fasts and hunger strikes,[49] but to these transient manifestations, which are the most frequent or at least more spectacular, are added here and there some beginnings of regular practices of fasting.

Certain permanent evils of our time indeed call for a permanent reaction, which seeks expression in fasting. The arms race has thus aroused not only the well-known sporadic manifestations, but also resolutions to fast once a week, for twenty-four or even thirty-six hours.[50] Similarly the hunger prevailing in a great part of the human race has drawn some Christians of the rich countries to deprive themselves of one meal a week, whose cost is then given to some charity for the underfed.[51] In this last case, the fast is intimately linked to its cause, and it obtains a true sympathy, in the strong sense of the word, with those who suffer. It is then less a public

49. P. Toulat, "Jeûnes publics et grèves de la faim," in *Christus* 29 (1982), pp. 196–200.

50. Pyronnet, "Le jeûne. Vivre d'amour et d'eau fraîche," in *Tychique* 45 (September 1983), pp. 19–26 (see p. 22: examples of Anglican and Catholic bishops in the United States).

51. P. Warlomont, "Avoir faim, geste actuel," in *Christus* 29 (1982), p. 187–189.

protest than a personal awakening of consciousness and of solidarity in action.

Conclusion: For a Typology of Fasting

However rapid, this survey has set before us a number of "fasts," varying in their durations, motives and modalities.

The fast can consist of not eating anything for a half-day, for one day (which might be called the "basic fast"), two days ("prolonged fast") and so on, up to forty days or until death. It can also consist of small, successive twenty-four hour fasts, each day having just one meal taken at a more or less late hour ("repeated fast"), for a limited or unlimited period. Or it can consist of eating only every two, three, four or five days (a prolonged and repeated fast), and is practiced more or less permanently. At the elementary level it can consist of a meal skipped, delayed or diminished. The differences between these forms of the "fast" are so great that one should never use the word without immediately specifying what one means.

There are also occasional fasts without any fixed period of recurrence, and programmed fasts inscribed on the calendar. Their different relation to time is usually accompanied by different aims, the first type responding to unforeseeable events, the second commemorating past events or spanning some cycle of time.

Both types can have many meanings: a person fasts as a sign of mourning or of desolation, of penitence or of supplication, but also with the aim of curing one's body or soul, to protest against injustice or to impress public opinion. Whether the fast is religious or simply natural, ascetic, medicinal or political, the fast is sometimes strictly private, indeed secret (think of Christ's recommendations, Mt 6:16–18); sometimes it has a social bearing or even a social plan, whether it be done by individuals or by groups.

The variety of modes is no less great, because fasting, essentially a matter of time, is complicated by rationing and abstinence, quantitative or qualitative privations, which are infinitely various. In addition, it makes a difference to fast without doing anything or while working, in an ordinary social milieu or in an especially appropriate one, with or without accompanying spiritual exercises such as scriptural meditation, and with or without the two evangelical concomitants of fasting: almsgiving and prayer (Mt 6:2–18).

So many distinct practices, motives and effects make an extremely rich environment for the "regular fast." By considering them we doubtless see better, first, what a small thing it is and all that it is not; but we also discover its affinities with many other forms of fasting. Whether by contrast or by analogy, these latter will help us better to understand and appreciate it.

CHAPTER III

The Birth and Significance of a Practice

NOW THAT I have defined the regular fast and tried to locate it in the world of related practices, I feel I have not yet finished with history. I must ask about the origin and meaning of this observance that comes from ancient monasticism. My personal experience of the fast is one thing, but the objective end of this act is something else. Without denying the former, I must first question the tradition that guides me, in order to understand how and why it has elaborated this rule.

The first step in the inquiry will consist in finding the most ancient signs of the observance of the regular fast in cenobitic monasteries. From there I shall try to ascend to the origins, either eremitical or secular, of this practice. Then I shall follow its evolution in the monasteries of the West for a century and a half, until St. Benedict. Finally I shall attempt to throw light on the meaning of the observance as it stands out in the texts we will have covered.

The First Witnesses

Strangely enough, it is not at the very origins of cenobitism but three-quarters of a century later, around the year 400, that we hear of the daily fast in monastic communities, many of whom, it is true, must have been practicing it for some time. In the first cenobitic grouping, that of St. Pachomius in upper Egypt about 325, the monks fasted only on Wednesdays and Fridays,[1] that is, on the two days of the "station" observed by the whole church, as we have seen. On the other days a signal resounded at midday for the common meal, and a second meal was prepared in the evening "for those who were fatigued, the old men and children, and during very hot weather." But this motivation already indicates that the second meal was a sort of anomaly, which is confirmed by the continuation of the text: Some eat hardly anything the second time; others are content with but one meal, either lunch (*prandii*) or dinner (*coenae*); some eat a little bread and leave. The meal is taken in common; he who does not wish to come to the refectory receives in his cell only bread, water and salt, either for one day or for two days if he prefers.

Pachomian monasticism, while not exceeding in principle the ordinary fast of Christians, was thus influenced by an ascetic tendency that went far beyond it. It is this tendency that will express itself in the testimony at the end of the century when the community regime itself will impose a daily fast on everyone.

1. Jerome, "Preface to the Rule of St. Pachomius," 5 (see below, note 6). Cf. *Precepts* 90 (at least in the Coptic) and 103: "noon"; 111 and 115: "the two fasts." *Pachomian Koinonia*, vol. 2, Cistercian Studies 46, p. 141ff. (Kalamazoo, MI: Cistercian Publications, 1981).

The Cenobites of Egypt and of Gaul

The first of these texts in time is the famous description of the cenobites in Egypt, inserted by Jerome in 384 in his letter to Eustochium.[2] He describes these monks as enclosed in their cells from morning until the middle of the afternoon (the ninth hour). Then they gather to pray and to hear a conference by the superior. This conference is followed by the meal, which is therefore taken sometime after None. At the meal is served "bread, dry vegetables and green vegetables, with seasoning of salt and oil," wine being reserved for the old men. These latter, together with the children, often have the right to a lunch as well. A little further on, Jerome notes that "the fast is uniform all year," except for Lent, the only time when one is permitted to do more. During the fifty days of Easter time the monks are content to advance the one meal by three hours. This midday meal thus becomes "a lunch" (*prandium*) and is considered to satisfy the Church's tradition that forbids fasting during the fifty days. The monks thus avoid overloading their stomachs by taking two meals.

At the same time in the remotest part of Gaul, the eighty monks gathered around St. Martin of Tours seem to have done about the same. Sulpicius Severus, writing around the year 397 evoked this community of Marmoutier, saying that "all took their meal together after the hour for the fast."[3] The

2. Jerome, *Epistles* 22, 35.
3. *Life of St. Martin* 10,7.

community meal thus took place at the ninth hour at the earliest, and did so every day, it seems.

The Ordo monasterii *and Cassian*

A little set of regulations traditionally annexed to the Rule of St. Augustine and called the *Ordo monasterii*, witnesses more precisely to the daily fast until the ninth hour, at least five days out of seven. This document, which doubtless emerged in North Africa around the year 395, prescribes manual work until noon, and then reading for three hours. "At the ninth hour they return the books" and eat their meal.[4]

For a long time this horarium left me pensive. I could scarcely imagine these monks reading profitably at the hottest hour of the day, with an empty stomach since waking, after six hours of manual work under the African sun. Everything seemed to combine to make these hours of reading fruitless. Today, my experience of fasting enables me to understand all that. Far from being the empty period I imagined, the hours preceding the meal are the best of the day, when the mind is most lucid and the body most vigorous. Very wisely, the author of the *Ordo* reserved this choice moment for reading.

Thus the spiritual meal, taken under the best conditions, precedes the bodily meal. Similarly, as we have just seen, the Egyptian cenobites described by Jerome listened to the superior's conference just before going to the refectory. This

4. *Ordo monasterii* 3; cf. 7 (Wine).

priority given to the soul's nourishment corresponds to an old monastic instinct, a trace of which survives even today in the custom of listening to some sentences of the refectory book before unfolding one's napkin. But apart from this simple recognition of the primacy of the spiritual, it is in the present case a wise use of time, devoting to the hearing of the word of God the hours when man is best disposed to receive it.

Before leaving the *Ordo monasterii*, we should note that this laconic text shows us that on Saturday the monks were dispensed from fasting. On that day as well as on Sunday the brothers could drink wine. The assimilation of Saturday to Sunday was general in the East, where the *Ordo* seems to have its roots. When Cassian, writing about the year 425, reports in his *Institutes* his memories of those regions, going back about forty years, he remarks that the cenobites there do not fast on Saturday and Sunday. On those days they dine at midday and a second optional meal is prepared for them in the evening.[5] Five days out of seven: this part of the week given to fasting should be compared with the exactly inverse proportion we met with among the Pachomians. They observed only the traditional "stations" of Wednesday and Friday, being in principle dispensed from fasting the other five days. The few decades separating Pachomius from Cassian and the *Ordo monasterii* thus saw a complete

5. Cassian, *Institutes* 3, 9–12.

reversal—at least in appearance, for we remember that Pachomius' monks did not seem to pay much heed to the facilities offered to them,[6] an attitude that we find elsewhere in Cassian's cenobites in regard to dinner on feast days.

The Rule of the Four Fathers

One last witness remains to be heard: the third of the "Four Fathers," decked out with Egyptian pseudonyms, who composed the first rule of the monastery of Lerins around 400–410. We owe to this Paphnutius (who was perhaps St. Honoratus, the founder of Lerins) a time schedule that is all the more interesting in that it includes a scriptural justification. This biblical motive, although seemingly obscure, is precious nonetheless, for it is the first we encounter in these documents so inexplicit and full of dry regulations.

When the *Rule of the Four Fathers* comes to the question of fasting, it begins by invoking a scriptural text: "Peter and John were going up to the temple at the hour of prayer, at the ninth hour (three o'clock in the afternoon)" (Acts 3:1). And it concludes: "Therefore we must observe this rule, never to eat in the monastery before the ninth hour, except on Sunday."[7] This reasoning leaves us perplexed, for we scarcely

6. According to a text of Jerome (preface of his translation of the *Rule of Pachomius*) which dates only from 404. Was this ascetic fervor already vigorous in Pachomius' time?

7. "Rule of the Four Fathers," 3, 2–5. *Early Monastic Rules* (Collegeville, MN: The Liturgical Press, 1982), p. 25.

see the connection between the text of Acts dealing with an hour of prayer, and the observance of the fast that claims to be based on it. But Tertullian's book *De ieiunio* mentioned above, furnishes us with the key to this singular type of argument. In it we see indeed that this passage of Acts, already in the third century, was considered as a testimony about fasting. Peter and John, it was thought, were going to pray at the ninth hour before taking their meal. Tertullian rightly contests this exegesis, but he attests that it was current and even had normative value among the Catholic faithful, who based on it their custom of ending the stational fast at the ninth hour.[8]

Two Historic Roots: The Station on Wednesdays and Fridays

The Fathers of Lerins, in referring to this phrase of St. Luke to justify the monks' daily fast, were therefore only taking advantage of a traditional interpretation. The relation thus established between the monks' daily fast and the "stations" of the ancient church deserves the closest attention. We no doubt have here one of the historical roots of the regular fast. The latter seems an extension of the stational fast, which has been made daily. The monks have decided to do every day what the Christians of the past centuries used to do twice a week.

8. Tertullian, *De ieiunio* 10 (cf. 2).

We can see a confirmation of this origin of the monastic fast in the fact that Cassian freely uses the word "station" to designate the late hour of the monks' meal. The ninth hour is when one "ends the station of the fast." Thus for the monks there is a "daily station" that is distinguished from the "obligatory station" of Wednesdays and Fridays, although Cassian sometimes also qualifies the daily station with the adjective "obligatory."[9] This application of the old word *statio* to the new reality of the daily fast shows that the latter was regarded as a prolongation of the former.

Such then, it seems, is the first root of the regular fast. We might qualify it "pre-monastic" or "secular"; the monks' own contribution was to make continuous the sporadic observance of ordinary Christians, by introducing it into daily living.

The daily fast of the hermits

The other root of the regular fast is to be sought among the hermits. Just as Judith before Christ and Anna in the very time of Jesus, so those other contemporaries of Christ, the *Therapeutae*, observed a daily fast according to Philo. And this fast did not end at the ninth hour, like that of the station. Only "after the set of sun," as we remember, did these Jewish ascetics take their very frugal nourishment: bread,

9. Cassian, *Conferences* 2, 25 and 21, 29, 2 (*statio ieiunii*); *Institutes* 5, 24 (*cotidiana statio... légitimée*) and 20 (*statio legitima*).

water and salt, made slightly more pleasant by hyssop for the more delicate. Still that was just the practice common to all, for some remained fasting for three or even six days.[10]

We might doubt that these exploits of the *Therapeutae* served as models for the Christian monks who were so little inclined to follow non-Biblical examples. But between Philo and the first Christian monastic writers one author had taken care to annex these Jewish precursors to Christianity. Eusebius of Caesarea in his *Ecclesiastical History*, written shortly before the end of the persecutions, presented the *Therapeutae* as the first believers in Alexandria, converted by the evangelist Mark, who would have surpassed in fervor the first faithful of Jerusalem described by St. Luke.[11]

Thus Christianized, these great Jewish fasters fascinated certain authors who recounted the first attempts at the regular fast by Christian monks, and perhaps they fascinated the monks themselves. When Athanasius reports the beginnings of Anthony's asceticism, he manifestly has Philo's account in mind. Anthony, he says, "ate once a day, after sunset. Sometimes he took food only after two days, often after even four days. And his sole nourishment was bread and salt, with water to drink."[12]

10. Philo, *De vita contemplativa* 34–35 and 37 (cf. above, Chapter II, note 16).
11. Eusebius, *Ecclesiastical History* 2, 17, 16–17.
12. Athanasius, *Life of Anthony* 7, 6.

This diet and the very language describing it resembles that of the *Therapeutae* too much for Athanasius to have been able to report it independently of Philo's text. At a distance of two or three centuries, Anthony thus appears as a descendant of the Jewish heroes. Among the few traits that distinguish him from his predecessors, we note that Athanasius did not dare to attribute to him fasts of three and six days, but only of two and four days.

A reduction of the same kind is observed in another passage of a Christian monastic author who borrows no less visibly and even explicitly from the picture given by Philo. When Cassian, at the beginning of the second book of his *Institutes*, tells of the origin of monasticism in Egypt, he shows us St. Mark's disciples eating only at the end of two or three days, and not before sunset.[13] The reduction, here more obvious than in Athanasius, is compensated for, however, by Cassian's passing over in silence the simple fast of one day, and presenting "two or three days" as the current norm of these first monks.

Whatever may be said about this rivalry, the present text of the Institutes is all the more important for the history of the regular fast in that it exists in a work meant for cenobites and claims to trace the origins of cenobitic monasticism. According to a myth that Cassian develops elsewhere,[14] the

13. *Institutes* 2, 5, 2.

14. *Conferences* 18, 5.

observance evolved in the first generations of the cenobitic movement in the West.

The facts

At the beginning, around the year 400, the daily fast until the ninth hour seems firmly established in Augustinian Africa, in the Gaul of Martin and the Provence of the Four Fathers. But a century and a half later the Rule of St. Benedict attests a serious yielding, at least in Italy. While the fast is maintained in winter and in Lent, it disappears not only in Easter time, when the monks take two meals each day, but also for five days out of seven in the summer. During that season the only fast days are Wednesdays and Fridays. Again, Benedict permits dining at noon even on those two days if the monks are working at the harvest or the heat becomes burdensome.[17] Some texts allow us to glimpse the vicissitudes of the regular fast between the first cenobitic rules and that of Benedict. About twenty years after the Four Fathers, the *Second Rule of Lerins* says nothing about the time of meals, but we cannot draw any conclusion from this silence because of the extreme brevity of the document. But at the end of the century, the so-called *Rule of Macarius*, which seems to have issued from the same Lerins milieu, sounds a disturbing note. In an appendix it declares that the Wednesday and Friday fast is inviolable under pain of grave

17. *Rule of St. Benedict* (RB) 41,1–7.

fault.[18] What about the other days? We are reduced to the ancient secular "stations," below the daily regime that the monks had made their norm.

What we conjecture by reading "Macarius" becomes obvious when we come to Caesarius of Arles. In his *Rule for Nuns* drawn up between 512 and 534, he no doubt shows himself a little more demanding than Benedict in maintaining once a week in Easter time the old principle of one meal: on that day, Friday, the nuns doubtless take only the one meal at noon time, just as Jerome's cenobites did every day in Easter time. But from Pentecost to September 1, Caesarius is still more prudent than the Benedictine rule: he abstains from prescribing anything and leaves everything to the abbess's decision. In addition, the winter fast itself is notably impaired: in September and October as well as from Epiphany to Sexagesima Sunday, the nuns fast only on Mondays, Wednesdays and Fridays. Thus the daily fast (not counting Saturdays) only continues to exist from November 1 to Christmas and the seven days before Epiphany.[19]

It is true that in his *Rule for Monks*, written between 534 and 542, Caesarius returns to stricter norms, men being

18. *Rule of Macarius* 29. (see note 7 above, p. 51). Cf. *Enquete sur les moines d'Egypte* 8, 58. English translation, Cistercian Studies 34, *The Lives of the Desert Fathers* (Kalamazoo, MI: Cistercian Publications, 1982), p. 78.

19. Caesarius, *Rule for Virgins* 66, 15 (Paschal time); 67, 1 (summer) and 2–5 (winter); *Rule for Monks* 22, 1.

thought stronger than women. But even there, the bishop of Arles is satisfied with the Wednesday and Friday fast for summertime. After him, the Provencal legislations that depend on him, that of Aurelian of Arles and that of the monastery of Tarnant, are no more demanding. The decline of the daily fast is therefore a general and definitive phenomenon. In both Gaul and Italy, the monks in summer fall back upon the twice weekly fast of the ancient church. Even this is not assured, for evasions are more or less explicitly provided for almost everywhere.

The interpretation of the facts

How was this general evolution, strangely leading the cenobitism of the sixth century to a sort of compromise between the Pachomian observance and that of the first Western rules, felt and judged by those who lived it? The Provencal rules tell us nothing, but the Italian rules give us glimpses. Just before Benedict, the *Rule of the Master*, which is Benedict's principal source, still maintains the ancient norms on almost every point: the daily fast until the ninth hour, even in summer; the single midday meal in Paschal time. But this fidelity to tradition was not accomplished without trouble. The Master felt himself obliged to justify the primitive observance, and the exceptions to which he consented in favor of certain brothers, that is, the sick, travelers, children and old men, foretold the general mitigation that was going to be practiced by Benedict. Beginning his plea for the ninth hour, the Master cried out: "Let us spiritual men blush at evading the fast until the ninth hour...."[20]

"To blush"—this word recurs under Benedict's pen in the Epilogue of his Rule.[21] Of course there he was not dealing explicitly with the fast, but the "blush of shame" that Benedict says he experiences in comparing the monks of his time to those of the past is no doubt motivated chiefly by the mitigation he knew he himself had made in this matter. Other signs confirm this, notably the sort of hesitant bad conscience with which he forces himself to compensate for the evident relaxation of the meal schedule with at least verbal restrictions in the matter of food and drink.

The abandonment of the daily fast in the sixth century seems then to have been felt as indeed a decline or as decadence. Of course, we today may think that the monastic legislators then proved their wisdom and realism, since the lessening of the summer fast with Benedict no doubt stemmed in large part from his authorization of field work, which the Master forbade. We might even find the new regime more satisfying than the old one, whose uniformity did not recognize the fact that in the ancient horarium based on the sun, the summer fast was much heavier to bear, because of the heat and the length of the day and the shortness of sleep. But it does not seem that St. Benedict and

20. *Rule of the Master* (RM) 28, 3.

21. RB 73, 7.

his contemporaries appreciated in the same way these merits that we are inclined to see in the mitigated regime. What struck these monks of the sixth century was rather the negative aspect of an evolution that weakened one of the essential characteristics of monasticism.

Why the Regular Fast?

This importance attributed to fasting among the components of the monastic life is precisely what remains for us to explain. What then was the meaning of this observance, judged to be so fundamental? To answer such a question one might survey, as I have done elsewhere,[22] the many and multiform patristic texts that treat fasting. But the concrete approach I have adopted here moves me to be content with the small number of indications furnished by the documents we have just encountered. These explicit or (very often) implicit motives, linked to the very practice of the cenobites, will make us penetrate more surely into the thought and heart of the fasting monk, than speculative expositions would.

---

22. *La Règle de saint Benot*, t. VII, "Commentaire doctrinal et spirituel," (Paris: Les Éditions du Cerf, 1977), p. 320–333. English translation, Cistercian Studies 54, p. 229–238.

Fasting, chastity, prayer

Perhaps the best way of entering into this psychology is to consider the two biblical prototypes of perpetual fasting: Judith and Anna. Without any theorizing, these two women impose the idea of an indissoluble bond uniting fasting with chastity and prayer, at the center of a life consecrated to God. It is not a matter of this or that particular effect of the fast, but of the seal imprinted on one's entire being by submitting the most imperious of the bodily appetites to religious discipline.

Fasting and chastity are inseparable, for the oblation of the sexual instinct does not succeed without that of the eating instinct. Fasting and prayer are inseparable, for the raising of the soul towards God does not succeed without detachment from created things. Although we can and should pray without ceasing, even with a full stomach, the soul is much more free to go to God when it is not absorbed with digestion.

I have just referred to the words of St. Paul and of Christ himself, "Pray without ceasing," the watchword that dominates the whole ascesis of monks and focuses their desire.[23] If fasting is the natural associate of prayer, it should in its own way have the same character of perpetuity. As the monk knows he is invited to pray without ceasing, so he feels himself called to practice fasting not transiently, but habitually.

23. Thess 5:17; Lk 18:1. Cf. Cassian, *Conferences* 9, 2, 1.

In this perspective we understand that Lent, the chief time for prayer and fasting, seems like the symbol and summary of the monastic life: "The life of a monk ought to be a continuous Lent" says St. Benedict.[24] The continual fast, which is more effective during these forty days than at any other time, should thus seem the ideal norm for the monk. The whole monastic life, as a preparation for the eternal Easter, should be marked with this sign.

Monasticism is essentially a search for unity. It does not thrive on distinctions and divisions. That is why the occasional or discontinuous fast is less natural to it than the regular, or indeed, perpetual fast.

Fasting and almsgiving

This character of simplicity and totality, which tends to unify the monk's life in fasting and in prayer, appears also in another connected domain, that of alms. This comes to mind as soon as we speak of fasting and praying, since it appears in company with these two holy works, indeed before them, in the Sermon on the Mount.[25] But just as the monk tends to fast every day and to pray at every moment, so he practices almsgiving not in a partial but a total way: "Go, sell what you possess and give it to the poor." Whether the monk gives his heart in prayer, or his material body in

24. RB 49, 1.
25. Mt 6:2–4 (alms); 5–15 (prayer); 16–18 (fasting).

fasting, or his material goods in alms, the three great religious acts of the Gospel are invested for him with the same aspect of an offering without reserve, each in its own way.

Fasting and almsgiving are thus related by their common character of a Gospel work pushed to the limit, and they are still more closely united by a true relation of cause to effect: fasting demands and makes possible generosity towards the other. Third Isaiah insists that the fast be accompanied by acts of justice and goodness.[26] But with Christians the relation becomes still stricter: what one deprives oneself of by fasting is given in alms. As early as the middle of the second century, one of the most ancient writings of Christianity, *The Shepherd* of Hermas, lays down this rule that sounds so modern: on fast days let the Christian be content with bread and water, calculating the money thus saved and giving it as a gift to the poor.[27] The Jewish *Therapeutae*'s meal on bread and water thus takes on a social meaning; self-imposed privation becomes a source of charity. While in the Church some bishops like St. Leo the Great insisted on this charitable aspect of fasting, the monks did not neglect it. Cassian, without establishing an explicit relationship between the two facts, notes in turn the extreme detachment of the Egyptian cenobites

26. Is 58:3–10.

27. Hermas, *The Shepherd* 56, 7. For a prescription inserted at a later date, for the intention of the monks, in an apophthegm, see L. Régnault, *Les Sentences des Pères du désert. Série des Anonymes* (Solesmes-Bellefontaine, 1985), p. 317, no. 1741.

and their extraordinary generosity. On the one hand, each was permanently content with one pound of bread a day, although his work earned him much more. On the other hand, the monasteries shipped cargoes of foodstuffs to the prisoners in the nearby cities and to populations in the impoverished regions around them.[28] It is obvious that these monks could show such generosity because they refused to better their lot as they could easily have done.

This witness of Cassian's about Egyptian monasticism is confirmed by several contemporary authors and aroused an echo in the Latin West. When the Master and St. Benedict in the spiritual part of their Rules enumerate the maxims that should control the monks' behavior, the famous "instruments of good works," they juxtapose "To love fasting" and "To relieve the poor."[29] That this sequence does indeed signify a causal relationship is proved by the literary source of the passage, a passion of a martyr where a phrase "in view of..." joins the two maxims. The monks impose the restrictions of fasting on themselves, at least in part, to be able to feed the needy.

The Master being more picturesque and detailed than Benedict, illustrates this relationship of the fast and almsgiving by a charming prescription:

---

28. Cassian, *Institutes* 4, 14 and 10, 22.

29. RM 3, 13–14; RB 4, 13–14. Cf. *Passio Iuliani* 46.

> Should one of the disciples wish to turn down part of the regular measure of drink or the bread he has left over...when the abstinent brother turns this down, let him say in a low voice to the cellarer clearing the table: "Take this too, and may what is denied the flesh redound to God." Then the cellarer puts this into a separate container to redound abundantly to God, and lets it be added as a gift to the monastery's alms and given by the cellarer into the hand of a poor beggar.[30]

Fasting as ascesis

The connection between renunciation and charity, so dear to present-day Christianity, is therefore not at all alien to the monastic thought of antiquity. However, we would be wrong to insist on it too much, for the monks' fast obviously has other and deeper motives. In the passage I have just cited, the Master chiefly congratulates the abstinent brother for showing himself "as someone who loves the spirit more than the flesh, by putting the curb of chastity on lust." After having noted the relationship of fasting with almsgiving in line with the Sermon on the Mount, it is time for us to consider the properly ascetic aspect of fasting, which is of primordial importance.

30. RM 27, 47–51.

For this we have a good guide in the person of Philo, witness of the monastic fast among the Jews and inspirer of its practice among the Christians. Philo immediately places the *Therapeutae's* fast under the sign of temperance (*egkrateia*). This latter, he says, is for them "like the foundation of the soul that they lay first in order to build the other virtues on it." Then he traces the program of dietary restrictions that we have seen. Temperance, therefore, is the fundamental virtue of the monk, and it finds its most immediate expression in the control of the desire to drink and eat, before the simplification of one's dwelling place and clothing.

When we pass from this page of Philo's to that of Athanasius (see note 12) who was inspired by it, we find the same theme, but Christianized by a reference to the Apostle Paul. After a series of impure temptations, over which he triumphed by the grace of God, Anthony understood that the devil would not cease attacking him, and that as a result he must constantly be on guard. He found the watchword for this continual "ascesis" in Paul's saying: "I punish my body and subdue it" (1 Cor 9:27). Fasting appears then as one means of subduing the body, along with other practices such as watchings, sleeping on a hard bed, and renouncing the use of oil for anointing the body. We might even say that fasting is the means par excellence. When a Christian of that era remembered St. Paul's words, he automatically and almost exclusively thought of privations of food: almost every one of the dozens of citations of 1 Cor 9:27 refers to fasting. The

Master and St. Benedict, among many others, are witnesses of this spontaneous interpretation. In their "Instruments of Good Works" the recommendation of fasting, "To love fasting," is introduced by a reminder of the Pauline maxim, whose obvious purpose is to lay the foundation and mark the Christian meaning of fasting: "To punish the body."[31]

Temperance, ascesis, subjection of the body—call it what you like—such is indeed the essential purpose of fasting and the incomparable service it renders man. Philo and Athanasius, each in his own way, refer to the astonishing flight of the spirit that results from this right conditioning of bodily appetites. For the Jewish thinker, fasting is accompanied by intense spiritual activity. All day long the *Therapeutae* "philosophized," that is, they read and interpreted scripture. Their daring escapes from the daily necessity of eating are provoked by a veritable passion for religious knowledge, as if the hunger for contemplation developed in inverse proportion to the hunger for eating.

Athanasius is more sober, but he also notes a relation of inverse proportionality between the vigor of the superior faculties and the vivacity of sense pleasures. To weaken the latter is to strengthen the former. And he cites another saying of the Apostle: "for whenever I am weak, then I am strong" (2 Cor. 12:10). The citation may appear more or less

31. RM 3, 11, *corpus pro anima castigare* (to punish the body for the sake of the soul)—RB 4, 11, *corpus castigare* (to punish the body).

commonplace, but the anthropology it claims to illustrate affords matter for reflection. That bodily mortification is a demand of the Spirit and a condition for spiritual expansion is what many passages of Paul seem to affirm, and in any case the primitive ascetic tradition, continued by monasticism, unanimously bears witness to the same. My own experience of fasting, however limited it may be, allows me fully to verify this law.

Two Scriptural foundations of the fast

To return to the text of 1 Corinthians which Athanasius uses as a watchword for Anthony's whole ascetic program, "I punish my body and subdue it," we can say that by its constant application to fasting in patristic literature it constitutes the chief scriptural foundation of this practice, considered from the ascetical point of view. But there is another New Testament word that plays an important role in this domain, showing a different aspect of fasting. It is Jesus' word reported with slight variant by the three Synoptic Gospels: "The wedding guests cannot mourn as long as the bridegroom is with them, can they? The days will come when the bridegroom is taken away from them, and then they will fast."[32]

The great interest of this Gospel word lies in its putting the fast in direct relation to the person of Christ. And not

32. Mt 9:15; Mk 2:9–20; Lk 5:34–35. Cf. above, Chapter II, note 19.

only the fast, but also its opposite: the dispensation from the fast, indeed the prohibition of the fast. Under this last aspect this Gospel word is cited by Cassian in a Conference that treats precisely "Of the Remission (of the fast) during Easter time."[33] Indeed it is a law of the Church, confirmed by monasticism, that no one fasts on the days when we specially celebrate Christ risen and newly present among the living, whether it be the weekly Sunday or the fifty days of Easter time each year. And since Christ is present in each of our brother Christians or monks—"You have seen your brother, you have seen the Lord"—monasticism very logically applied the word to the religious event constituted for the monk or monastery by the arrival of a guest. Again Cassian notes the fact: when we receive the visit of a guest, the fast must be suspended in his honor, because the Bridegroom is there.[34]

Thus the interruption of the fast appears as a sign of Christ's presence, and correlatively, the fast is connected with his absence. And this not only on the days when we specially remember his disappearance, such as the Wednesdays and Fridays of each week and the days before Easter each year, but also during the whole lapse of time that precedes his second coming. Certainly Christ is indeed present to us all during the centuries of our Christian history, since

33. Cassian, *Conferences* 21, 18, 2.

34. Cassian, *Institutes* 5, 24 (cf. *Conferences* 21, 18, 2).

he lives and we live by his life. But no less really is he absent, since he remains invisible and like a stranger to our sensible world.

This permanent absence of Christ lays the foundation of the regular fast. Besides the feast days when the Church recalls the meeting with Christ at Easter and anticipates the meeting at the Parousia, the whole of Christian time is marked by the remoteness of the Bridegroom, the wait for his coming, and consequently by fasting. The monk's habitual solitude is also added to this absence of Christ: the Lord's visits under the appearances of a guest only interrupt transiently a normal state of separation.

Paul's word—"I punish my body"—and Jesus's word—"When the bridegroom is taken away from them"—place the Christian fast therefore in two very different lights. The first shows its ascetic aim, for the good of the faster himself. The second defines it in relation to another person: Christ. In the first perspective the present life is considered as a time of struggle and effort, in which man, divided and disordered, seeks to reconquer his interior unity and order. In the second, life appears as a time of separation during which we aspire to see Christ and to enter into his kingdom. In the first case the abstention from food aims at disciplining the appetite by reducing it to strict necessity. In the second, it looks toward the coming of Christ as if the animal act of eating, egoist in itself, called for the presence of a friend in order to become communion.

The place of the fast in Christianity according to Cassian

Supported by these two scriptural roots, the fast is solidly joined with the perfect Christian life such as the monks want their life to be. Perhaps no one has emphasized more strongly than John Cassian that the monastic life demands habitual fasting. Rereading some pages of this great author is no doubt the best way to succeed in penetrating the spirit of the regular fast.

Cassian's fifth Conference gives fasting a significant place, at the very beginning of the ascetic effort and the pilgrimage towards the Promised Land. Cassian there treats "the eight principal vices" catalogued by his master Evagrius. The first of these is *gula*, that is, the disorderly appetite for eating. While he relates the seven following vices, from lust to pride, with the seven nations of Canaan dispossessed by Israel under Joshua, Cassian identifies *gula* with Egypt, the land from which the Chosen People had first to depart in order to undertake the struggle against these nations.

In other words, the discipline of fasting is man's first step in pursuit of perfection. This "departure from Egypt" precedes and conditions the whole effort of purification from the vices. The Christian and the monk must fast. To quit fasting is to return to Egypt.[35]

35. Cassian, *Conferences* 5, 18.

No less vigorous and suggestive under its mythical veneer is the pseudo-historical perspective of Conference 21. With the help of Eusebius' mistaken identity regarding Philo's *Therapeutae*, considered as the first Christians of Alexandria converted by St. Mark, Cassian, as we have seen, makes "the uniform fast all year long" a practice of the entire Church in the Apostolic era. He assures us that what the Christians of his era did in Lent, the first Christians did constantly. Lent with its thirty-six and a half days of fasting is only a tithe of the year. If there has been a passage from the totality of time to this fraction, it is because the Christian people quickly lost its first fervor, as proved by the decree of the Council of Jerusalem reported by St. Luke (Acts 15:28–29); the Apostles, to check this decadence, had to fix a minimum period during which at least once a year people would resume the spiritual effort of purification and of the service of God.[36]

In this myth of the origins of the Church, fasting accompanies the renunciation of property attested by the Acts of the Apostles. Both are the natural effects of the grace of Christ and the normal characteristics of a Christian. What the Old Law imposed in an obligatory and limited way, namely the payment of the tithe and the observance of the fast from time to time, the Spirit of Christ pushes Christians to accomplish spontaneously and without reserve: they abandon all their goods and they fast every day. This surpassing of the law by

36. Cassian, *Conferences* 21, 28–30.

voluntary devotion, influenced by a grace of detachment and unlimited love, is for Cassian the specific mark of the Gospel. To take back property rights and the possession of one's own goods is to return to the Old Testament, to lose Christian liberty and to fall again under the yoke of the Law.

The fast, thus associated with the evangelical counsel of poverty, is equally inseparable from the counsels of chastity and non-violence. Just as Christ invites him who wishes to be perfect to abandon all his goods, so he urges him to make himself a eunuch for the Kingdom of Heaven. And total chastity, affecting even the use of the eyes and reaching into the depths of the heart, is accompanied by love of one's enemies, the abandonment of revenge, nonresistance to wrongs suffered.[37] This ensemble of absolute and free gifts that characterize Christ's disciple, put the true Christian life beyond the letter of the law and every commandment, in the freedom of love and of the Spirit.

The fast is solidly connected with all that, in the regime of grace and the Gospel. In Cassian's eyes the monk's perpetual fast is one of those spontaneous offerings made by a man touched by Christ's grace and moved by the Spirit. As an efficacious sign of detachment from the world and attachment to God alone, it is part of the condition of regenerated man, on his march towards the Kingdom.

37. Mt 19:12 and 5:27–30 (chastity); 5:38–48 (non-violence). Cassian, *Conferences* 21, 33, 2–3 (chastity); 3–5 (poverty); 6 (non-violence).

These views of a fifth-century theoretician of the monastic life may seem questionable on many points in the eyes of a more modern exegesis and theology. Their value is nonetheless great for reconstituting the atmosphere in which the practice of the regular fast developed. As an heir of this practice, I am grateful to Cassian for explaining to me what it meant for the Fathers who established it. On this point as on many others, without hiding the problematic elements of such theories, I receive them as a light on my vocation, which is to follow Christ in the wake of the Fathers, listening to the word of God with an ear attuned to theirs. I love to know that this practice of the regular fast, whose benefits I experience, is linked in the minds of those who instituted it with the great evangelical renunciations that constitute Christ's disciple.

CHAPTER IV

Stages and Causes of the Decline

The absence of fasting among the monks of today

Of all the communities of monks, black or white, serving God today under the Benedictine Rule, there is, to my knowledge, not one that observes closely or remotely the horarium for meals fixed by St. Benedict. Instead of eating just one meal, at a more or less late hour, on fast days, that is, for more than half the year, and a maximum of two meals on the other days, the monks of our times grant themselves three meals every day that God makes, morning, noon and evening. Such is the massive and strange phenomenon on which I would like to reflect now. How and why has it come to pass that a fundamental observance of monasticism, duly codified by the Father of monks, has been tranquilly laid aside by the unanimous consent of his disciples?

The exception that makes the rule

However, scarcely have I written this word "unanimous" than there comes to mind a recent experiment which gives it the lie.

No, it is not entirely true that no Benedictine community practices the Rule in the matter of fasting. But the undertaking is so new, so isolated and still so frail that one scarcely dares to regard it as an institution having the promise of a long life.

At the end of a tour of the United States in 1984 I saw what I had never seen before: a group of men observing literally the Rule of St. Benedict. In the bottom of a canyon in New Mexico, at an altitude of more than six thousand five hundred feet, in a solitude separated from the smallest village by some twenty-five miles, a dozen men, young for the most part, were living joyously in extreme poverty, manual labor and the praise of God. Adobe huts in Indian style, furnishings that were less than sketchy, an absence of comfort and conveniences served as the framework of this life without compromise. The Liturgy of the Hours, sung in its entirety, has all the amplitude given it by the Rule, with a time of silent prayer after each psalm, according the custom of ancient monasticism.

The timetable for meals is also that of St. Benedict, which it sometimes even surpasses. During the month of November when I was visiting them, the monks were eating once a day, after the hour of None, around 4:30 P.M. I was told that those who needed to could have breakfast in the morning. The greater number waited for this one community meal.

But this is only an exception, as singular as it is beautiful. The general situation is as I have said, and it demands an explanation. Over the twenty or thirty years I have reflected on it, several causes have come to mind, without adequately explaining the phenomenon. I shall mention them first, before undertaking a new inquiry.

In Search of an Explanation

The enfeeblement of modern man?

The first explanation given me, and which I half-believed for several decades, is that of the diminution of human strength since antiquity. Today I believe, or rather I know by experience, that it is entirely false. I need not insist on the point, since I have said at the beginning of this essay how I have ascertained its falsity. If such a very ordinary man as I am experiences no difficulty in practicing the integral program of the Rule, and even going well beyond it, there is no doubt that this program remains within the capacity of modern man.

However, this myth of the enfeeblement of human health is very widespread and contributes powerfully to maintaining the present state of affairs. To the monks and their superiors, not to speak of the pastors of the Church and the Roman congregations, it offers a simple, obvious, reassuring justification of a practice which is really profoundly abnormal.

Work?

Even before I had proved to myself by experience the worthlessness of this explanation, the suspicions it aroused in me made me look in another direction. Guessing that we have just as much vigor as the Ancients, but that we employ it differently, I asked myself where the energy spent formerly on fasting was now being invested. It appeared probable to me that work had absorbed it and was preventing us from fasting today. In the disappearance of the fast I saw the sign and effect of a sort of collective extraversion: from the work on self, which is ascesis, we had passed to a work on things that was so exclusive and so demanding that it left no energy available for another effort.

This explanation was not as bad as the previous one, and no doubt contains some truth. In fact, work and the need for food go together. The "Master" to whom St. Benedict owes so much, forbade field work to his communities, because such labor would keep them from observing the fast. St. Benedict being obliged to admit certain types of agricultural labor, consequently mitigated the rule of fasting and granted some supplements.

What was true then is still true today. If all the monks do not work the land, far from it, it remains true that their intellectual or practical activities require a sufficient diet. In particular, for several decades work in the monasteries has taken on an increased importance, and tends to conform to the rhythm of modern work, with its well-known demands of regularity, output and comfort. A well-filled stomach seems to form part of these conditions of a relatively intense and profitable work, necessary both for the equilibrium of persons and the economic life of communities.

However, in repeating this explanation which I gave myself not long ago, I now perceive all its weakness.[1] For it is not true that the regular fast that I practice prevents working or even lessens the output. No doubt a more rigorous fast entailing rations less than the working man needed, would have this restraining effect. But there is no question of that. The Rule legislates for men who spend at least six hours a day in manual work. My regime, which goes well beyond what the Rule prescribes, has only developed my capacity to work. Provided that one takes a sufficient quantity of food at the one meal, the twenty-three hours preceding the next meal are fully available for work, the last hours of the daily cycle proving to be even the best by far. Since I have been waiting until evening to eat, my afternoons are much less heavy and tiring than when I took the noon meal.

This pretext of work is therefore scarcely less illusory than that of poor health, but, like the latter, it has taken hold of minds and acts strongly against any return to fasting. Especially in women's communities that have a hard time

1. Most recently in *The Rule of St. Benedict, A Doctrinal and Spiritual Commentary*, Cistercian Studies 54 (Kalamazoo, MI: Cistercian Publications, 1983), p. 230. A remark by Ph. Rouillard, "Jeûne," in *Catholicisme* 6 (1967), col. 833, says much the same thing.

earning their living and have rigorous work obligations, many superiors do not even want to hear of what they consider, for lack of personal experience, will likely weaken the sisters and imperil the subsistence of the monastery.

The common life?

After these two unsatisfying theories I must mention another one that was the fruit of my first experience of solitary life. In the first pages of this book I noted the relation between fasting and solitude. The man in solitude saves a large part of the energy spent in social life, and his energy so stored up is available for every kind of ascetic effort, and for fasting in particular. We might ask therefore if the incapacity to fast experienced by modern monks does not stem in large measure from the intensity of their communitarian life, which has only increased, since the Council, with the development of fraternal relations and the increase of "dialogue."

Here again the testimony of the Ancients is enlightening. In the very heart of the solitary life, one great monk experienced a sort of incompatibility between exchanges with another person and fasting. The admirable mystical author of the seventh century, Isaac of Niniveh, passes on to us this observation, which could well be a confidence on his part: One monk among the Fathers ate only twice a week. He told us: "On the days when I speak to someone, I cannot observe the fasting rule according to my custom, but I am obliged to break the fast."[2] He concludes that "the guard over the tongue...secretly contributes the vigor to accomplish the manifest works done by the body."

An analogous experience is reported in a text attributed to the same Isaac, but which seems really to pertain to a later Syrian author, John Saba of Dalyatha, in the eighth century:

> One Father told me...: "Every time I have relations with others, I eat three or four biscuits a day.... But when I separate from others to live in hesychia (silence, solitude, contemplation), the first day I eat one biscuit and a half, the second day just one biscuit. Then when my mind is deep in hesychia, I force myself to eat one whole biscuit, and I cannot.... But if someone comes to talk to me if only for an hour, it is impossible not to add something to my food and thus fail in my rule."[3]

From this it seems as if relations with one's neighbor, and conversations in particular diminish the self-mastery needed

---

2. Isaac of Niniveh, *Oeuvres spirituelles*, translated from the Greek by J. Touraille (Desclée de Brouwer, 1981), p. 71 (Discourse 3). The same statement exists in the Syriac text. See Isaac of Nineveh, *Mystic Treatises*, translated by A. J. Wensinck (Amsterdam, 1923), p. 260 (389 Bedjan).
3. Isaac of Niniveh, *Oeuvres spirituelles*, p. 249 (Discourse 43). This text is missing in the Syriac text translated by Wensinck. Inversely, the correlation between eating and talking is shrewdly noted by Gregory the Great, *Moralia* 1, 11: "Banquets almost always provoke talkativeness, and while the stomach fills, the tongue is loosened."

to remain fasting. We might add that the community celebration of the Divine Office has sometimes been felt as a fatiguing work that excused from fasting. Catherine de Bar (Mother Mechtilde of the Blessed Sacrament) who founded the Benedictines of Perpetual Adoration in the seventeenth century, learned one day that the sisters at her Rouen foundation were having trouble singing the Divine Office. She promised them she would send them the reinforcement of a strong voice at the first opportunity; meanwhile, everyone was dispensed from the regular fast. Two other letters confirm the gravity of the problem.[4] The choral office, conceived as an external work that must be accomplished with a certain decorum, cost what it may, absorbed a large part of the available energy, at the expense of this other essential element of monastic life, ascesis.

Thus the word seems to be an obstacle to fasting, whether one sings to the Lord or speaks to men. However little the expenditure of energy involved is increased, monks and nuns will find it difficult to maintain the restrictions on their diet. That is doubtless one of the reasons for the slow decline of fasting down the ages and its disappearance in our times.

Moreover, while the word constitutes the chief means of exchange between persons, it is only one of the elements of social life that compete with the effort to fast. Everything

4. Catherine de Bar, *Non date tregua a Dio. Lettere alle monache 1641–1697* (Milan, 1979), Jaca Book 49, p. 155–156 and 170.

in community life consumes energy. The constant necessity of being on time, of conforming to those around us, paying attention to our neighbors and supporting them, avoiding or dissipating the tensions with others, impose a constant constraint that costs energy. For that reason it is understandable that cenobites have always had more abundant fare than the hermits. This difference does not flow only from numbers and the obligation to take the weak into account. It is linked with the weight of the common life that the hermit does not undertake. If pushed to the limit, does not this burden become a true impediment for one who would wish to fast?

However, I fear that we are still quite far from the explanation we seek. Community life certainly does not suffice to account for our incapacity to fast. The proof is the fact that the fast regulated by St. Benedict is indeed meant for men living in community. Even today this fast proves practical not only for solitaries like me, but also for the cenobites of New Mexico of whom I just spoke, who moreover do not observe a particularly rigorous silence. I will add that, according to my experience, the very moderate fast envisaged by the Rule is certainly not helped by contacts and conversations, but they do not make it at all impossible. With a little practice a person observes the fast without trouble on days when he receives a visit or even gives a conference.

Search for other causes

While remembering that a certain way of living the community life can militate against fasting, we must reject the explanation that the disappearance of fasting is caused by the mere practice of community life. The cause of the phenomenon is still to be found.

A thorough study of the documents marking the evolution of monastic observances from the early Middle Ages until our day would be necessary to trace the stages of this progressive collapse of the fast and the motives evoked or implicit in each case. While not providing this study, I would at least like to survey very generally these fourteen centuries, dwelling on a few well-known facts and considering not only the observances of monasteries but also the general law of the Church and the practice of the faithful. At first glance it is indeed apparent that the monks and the Christian people have followed parallel paths, which end up about the same time in our day, with the same result. While granting a certain austerity proper to monks, the two evolutions are solidly connected and probably result from analogous causes.

The Evolution in the Church of the West

Since the evolution consists globally in the passage from a single meal taken at the end of the day, to two (noon and evening), then to three meals (with the addition of breakfast), several facts have to be considered. First, the advancement of the time of the sole or principal meal, which was progressively displaced from the evening to the middle of the afternoon and to the end of the morning. Then the addition of a secondary meal, the "collation," which took the place of the first meal at the end of day. Finally the appearance of breakfast in the early hours of the morning.

The anticipation of the meal

From the fifth to the eighth century, monks and faithful did not eat until evening during Lent. One of the first facts telling of a decline is the famous example of Charlemagne, who took his meal at the ninth hour (about 3:00 P.M.), invoking the necessities of etiquette.[5] The dignitaries who served him at table were themselves served later by lesser dignitaries, the latter in their turn by other inferiors. These successive meals of servants eating after their superiors stretched out in a line all afternoon and evening and the early part of the night, with the last ones sitting down to table only about midnight. The emperor therefore considered it a duty not to make his subjects wait too long and he anticipated the time of the

5. Reported by L. Thomassin, *Traité des jeûnes de l'Eglise* (Paris, 1700), 2nd ed., pp. 349–350. Unless otherwise noted, the facts mentioned below are borrowed from this work, as well as from E. Vacandard, "Carême," *Dictionnaire de théologie catholique* 2 (1905), col. 1724–1750.

meal for himself, not without having celebrated the office of Vespers, which had to precede the evening meal.

This particular case resulted from a general tendency, as we see by certain episcopal reactions. In 797 Theodulf of Orleans made great efforts to keep the meal in the evening, opposing those who advanced it to None (the middle of the afternoon). The innovation gained ground, and a bishop at the end of the tenth century, Ratherius of Verona, held that the hour of None was lawful, and even preferable to evening. The custom of eating in the middle of the afternoon was thus established, or just about, from that time on.

In 1072 the Council of Rouen insisted on maintaining this "ninth hour," already threatened by new anticipations, by recalling the primitive evening hour. The latter remained theoretically the rule for all, faithful and religious, as St. Bernard recalls in a sermon, but the way of calculating the hours then, inherited from antiquity, allowed the evening period to be considered as beginning at the end of the ninth hour. From then on, the monks were probably the only ones really to observe the fast until evening, as we see for example in the *Customs of the Charterhouse* drawn up by Guigo around 1120.[6]

6. Guigues, *Coutumes de Chartreuse* (Paris: Les Editions du Cerf, 1984), Sources chrétiennes 313, p. 160 (3, 1), 164 (4, 12), 186 (11, 4), etc. Cf. *Aux sources de la vie carthusienne* (La Chartreuse, 1967), t. VI, p. 587: the evening meal was then eaten at about 4:00 P.M., which was considered the end of the day.

However, the hour of None, canonized by the scholastic theologians and by St. Thomas Aquinas in particular, was not long in yielding as had the evening hour. At the end of the thirteenth century, the Franciscan Richard of Middleton extolled the sixth hour (midday), and the doctors after him were of the same opinion. Since the old principle of the evening meal remained in force, people continued to celebrate the office of Vespers before eating. From this arose the liturgical aberration that I still saw practiced in my first years in the monastery: Vespers was chanted before noon all during Lent. At least there was recognition that the real hour of the meal anticipated the normal hour, which remained what it was at the beginning.

At the end of the seventeenth century, certain individuals and even some religious communities did not hesitate to take their meal before noon even during Lent. The Oratorian Louis Thomassin, who states this fact without pleasure, sketches in this regard, with sharpness and humor, the mechanism of the long evolution by which the Lenten meal passed gradually from evening to midday and even into the morning hours:

> Apparently the same thing happened formerly to the hours of Vespers and of None, when the end of the fast was set there, as we see happening to the noon hour, by which the end of the fast is now determined. We can only determine the time for these

> things roughly, or about such and such an hour: *circa meridiem, circa horam nonam, aestimata hora vespera.* In consequence, by anticipating this hour a little, we do not seem to have done anything contrary to the rule of fasting. However, in the long course of years, by always advancing a little, it finally happened that around the year 1200 the office of Vespers and the end of the fast had been advanced from the evening hour to the ninth hour, and this change was made so imperceptibly that, when it was completed, even the learned did not even know that any change had been made. In the same way since the year 1200 when the offices of Vespers and the end of the fast had been fixed around the ninth hour, by always anticipating a little for two or three centuries and claiming it was always around the same time, they transferred and fixed Vespers and the Lenten meal about the noon hour in the year 1500. Since 1500 certain persons have anticipated the noon hour, claiming it was still around noon....[7]

Within this general movement that enveloped the whole church, what had the monks done in regard to the ecclesiastical fast and to their own regular fast? They acted doubtless

7. *Traité des jeûnes*, p. 360 (I have modernized the spelling). The chronological indications given here by Thomassin are notably later than those which I have indicated above according to the facts he himself alleges.

much more slowly than the faithful and their pastors, but they ended with about the same result.

In the second half of the thirteenth century a remark by Bernard Ayglier, abbot of Monte Cassino, in his commentary on the Rule, shows that the meal on fast days of the Rule continued to be taken about the hour of None.[8] But the Cassinese Declarations of 1680 put the meal at noon, both on days of the monastic fast and during Lent.[9] At the same period Abbot de Rancé himself showed himself no more rigorous:

> We go to the refectory on fast days of the Church, that is, during Advent and Lent, at 12:30 P.M.; on fast days of the Order, specially from the Exaltation of the Holy Cross, September 14, until Advent, at noon, and the rest of the time at 10:30 A.M.[10]

A century later, just before the Revolution, the Congregation of Saint Maur was at about the same point: the meal was at noon on the days of the ecclesiastical fast, and at 11:00 A.M. on the other days, including those of the regular fast.[11]

8. *In Regulam S. Benedicti Expositio* (Monte Cassino, 1894), p. 293.
9. *Regula S. Benedicti…cum Declarationibus Congregationis Casinensis* (Venice, 1723), p. 86 and 104.
10. *Règlements de la Trappe* (Paris, 1690), p. 118, cited by L. Dubois, *Histoire de l'Abbé de Rancé et de sa réforme*, t. 2; 2nd ed. (Paris, 1869), p. 87. The second edition of the *Règlements* (Paris, 1718), p. 15, says the same thing in different words.
11. *Regula S. P. Benedicti et Constitutiones Congregationis S. Mauri* (Paris, 1770), p. 127.

It was only at the Revolution, with the reform of Dom Augustine de Lestrange, that we see a decision made among the Trappists to conform strictly to the primitive Benedictine observances. The *Regulations* of La Val-Sainte have a flexible schedule in which "dinner" shifts from 11:30 A.M. or 12 noon (non-fast days) to 2:00 P.M. (regular fast days in summer), 2:30 P.M. (winter) and 4:15 P.M. (Lent).[12]

This regime was maintained, not without vicissitudes, for a century by one part of the Trappist monasteries, but it did not survive the 1892 reunion of the three Congregations issued from La Trappe. In all the monasteries today the monks eat at all seasons around noon almost invariably. Even the Carthusians have this fixed horarium characteristic of modern monasticism: winter or summer, whether a day of the regular fast or not, the first or only meal is taken at noon. In Lent it is delayed only by fifteen minutes.

The "collation" in the evening

The fast-day meal, by moving back from evening towards midday, left vacant its original place at the end of the day. The temptation to eat something at that time had to occur, and it did occur. When it was yielded to, a second element of the fast, and the most important one, disappeared: instead of only one meal a day, there were two.

---

12. *Réglemens... de Notre-Dame de la Trappe* (Fribourg, 1794) (1795 in fact), t. 2, pp. 7–23.

The abandonment of the principle of just one meal, which is the essence of the fast, seems to have occurred earlier in the East than in the West. In the middle of the eleventh century, Cardinal Humbert, spokesman of the Roman Church, reproached the Greeks for it, while boasting of the fidelity of the Latins. The Greeks, he said, allow themselves a second meal "of fruits and herbs." Even though it was light, this solid food taken outside the sole meal seemed scandalous to a Westerner.

I deliberately said "solid food," because drinking some liquid had long been authorized for fast-day evenings. In the sixth century the monks of the Roman region for whom the Rule of the Master was written, had a drink before going to bed when they had eaten at the ninth hour. During Lent when they ate in the evening, this last round of drinks was suppressed. However, the monastic council of Aix la Chapelle in 816 expressly authorized it for Lent. About the same time we hear of "fruits" being taken by the monks of certain Roman monasteries, along with the drink, during the reading before Compline,[13] but this laconic and little-known text, which merely declared they did thus "winter as well

13. *Ordo Romanus* 18, 8–9 (drawn up towards the end of the eighth century in Frankish territory). The gathering is called a *collecta*. The term *collatio*, which would eventually mean the small evening meal, derives from the fact that Cassian's *Conferences* (*Conlationes*) are the typical reading for this gathering before Compline, according to the Benedictine Rule (chapter 42). About the same time the *Ordo Cassinensis* II (*Ordo officii*) 8 states that the monks "eat a morsel" when they drink, after Vespers, on autumn days when the meal is at None.

as summer" does not envisage clearly enough the case of fast days, those of Lent in particular, for us to dare affirm the existence of such an early derogation to the rule of fasting. Moreover, was it proven, perhaps we should see therein a trace of the Greek influence on this Roman monastic milieu, where the Orientals were numerous during these centuries.

Whatever may be the truth about this exceptional witness, drinks at the end of the day were going to prove the effective opening wedge for a small meal of solid food during the following centuries. At the end of the thirteenth century St. Thomas Aquinas already admitted that joined to the drink were "electuaries," a sort of preserves that gave no cause for alarm both because of their inconsistency and their pharmaceutical character. Analogous products, still in semi-liquid or fondant form, remained in use in the last centuries of the Middle Ages under the name of "spices" until finally in the sixteenth century we hear of *cibus* (solid food) and bread. Taken at first in very small quantity—St. Charles Borromeo gave his people only an ounce and a half (forty-five grams)—this bread little by little gained in weight and other kinds of food were added. By the eighteenth century the level of eight ounces of food (close to two hundred fifty grams), including milk products and fish had been reached.

We see—notably by the example of the Carthusians—that the monks followed this evolution. In the middle of the fourteenth century, the Carthusians added the custom of drinking some wine on fast-day evenings, and at the end of the sixteenth century they allowed themselves in addition a piece of bread. This regime remains theirs today, although the collation remains optional and is not taken by all.[14]

Particularly significant in this matter are the vicissitudes of the Cistercian world, and of La Trappe in particular. In 1690, the *Regulations* of the Abbot de Rancé granted three ounces of bread (ninety grams) for collation on fast days of the Order, two ounces (sixty grams) on fast days of the Church.[15] But thirty years later, the second edition of the Regulations permitted only two ounces and one ounce respectively.[16] At the end of the century Dom Augustine de Lestrange completely removed this concession foreign to the Rule. With him, the primitive regime reappeared in all its purity for a hundred years: as with St. Benedict, the monk ate once a day, after None or after Vespers, and that was all. Finally, in 1892, Leo XIII put an end to this heroic

---

14. This information, as well as that concerning the present custom of Carthusians, I have from a Charterhouse in France. For the statutes of 1359 and 1580, see *Statuta* II, 4, 13; II, 10, 21.

15. *Règlements* (Paris, 1690), p. 132, cited by Dubois, *Histoire de l'Abbé de Rancé*, p. 87. According to Gervaise (manuscript of Port-du-Salut, p. 146–147; see note 17 below), this regime was established by Rancé only "two years after" the Lenten failure of 1673. The religious "treated it as a disgraceful relaxation and were constantly embarrassed by it."

16. *Règlements*, 2nd ed. (Paris, 1718). According to Gervaise, this regime was a return to that which Rancé had first fixed in 1673.

generosity, considered incompatible with the weakness of modern constitutions. The union of the three Trappist congregations obliged those who still maintained that regime to renounce it.

This long wandering journey of Rancé's sons in search of the lost fast is prefigured by the experience of the reformer of La Trappe himself. Twice, in 1672 and 1673, Rancé and his monks bravely attempted to practice Lent as prescribed by the Rule. The touching account of these attempts should be read in Abbé Dubois' *Histoire.* The religious of La Trappe, inflamed by the word of their superior, pressed him to take the last step separating them from the "summit of the Rule of St. Benedict," the great fast. At first hesitant, Rancé let himself be won over:

> It was resolved that the monks would observe the Lenten fast according to the terms of St. Benedict's Rule, that is, they would eat only one meal during this holy time, without a collation, about 4:00 P.M., after Vespers. This great austerity began on March 7, 1672. The Abbot had only allowed it as an experiment. He launched forth the first, like the eagle, with his eaglets following him in his sublime flight. They lasted about twenty-five days at this elevation. The bread was so coarse and heavy, the cider was so bad, the portions of vegetables so meager, the night vigils so long, the work so hard, the

psalmody so difficult, the air so unhealthy because of the exhalations from the ponds and small pools of water, their health was so weakened by the fevers that raged every autumn that their strength failed them. Soon it was impossible to maintain regularity with the few healthy religious who still remained on their feet, and it was with much difficulty that they made it to Easter.

This attempt would have been quite sufficient to discourage ordinary penitents; but these fervent disciples of St. Benedict were unwilling to admit defeat; they returned to the charge the following year to obtain a second Lent like the preceding one, hoping for more success. They even showed the desire to observe the regular fasts, especially from the Exaltation of the Holy Cross until Advent, with the same rigor as the fasts of the Church, except that they would take the single meal about 2:30 P.M., after the office of None.

Abbot de Rancé at first resisted for a long time; finally he decided to yield, and they began on All Saints Day of that year 1672. At the end of Lent in 1673 the ranks were still more depleted than in the previous year. The collapse was almost general. On Passion Sunday one-third of the members of the community were in the infirmary. Several others scarcely dragged themselves to the Office and to

> work like walking ghosts. Only about ten held out by the extraordinary vigor of their constitutions.[17]

According to the same book, these two failures made the reformer of La Trappe reflect and would explain the prudent horarium we see established by the *Regulations* of 1690.

We can smile at this tragi-comic page. But rather than its eighteenth-century style, touched up under Napoleon III, what I find savory is the substance of the tale. For one who knows how easy it is, even today, to observe the prescriptions of the Rule, there is something piquant in the spectacle of the first Trappists striving heroically and vainly to do something so simple. If they took such trouble and yet failed in the end, obviously they went about it in the wrong way.

Two major faults are apparent in their method. The chief one was lack of preparation: changing their regime suddenly, they underwent the insupportable shock of an austerity that one does not even perceive when one embraces it little by little. Then, there was the ruinous basis of the enterprise:

17. L. Dubois, *Histoire de l'Abbé de Rancé*, pp. 85–86. According to L. Lekai, "The Problem of the Authorship of De Rancé's 'Standard' Biography," in *Collectanea Cisterciensia* 21 (1959), pp. 157–163, this work is based on a biography written a century and a half earlier by the Trappist F. A. Gervaise, with Dubois merely renewing its presentation. Thanks to the kindness of the Father Librarian of Port-du-Salut, which preserves one of the two manuscripts of this unpublished *Life* (the text was revised by Dom Couturier, as was that of the "Sept Fons manuscript" cited by Dubois and now lost), I have been able to compare Gervaise and Dubois, who differs more from his model than Lekai allows us to suppose. Gervaise himself in this passage follows quite closely the Abbé de Marsollier, *La Vie de Dom A.-J. le Bouthillier de Rancé* (Paris, 1703), vol. 1, p. 331–333.

the inadequacy of the habitual diet and their poor state of health. If, instead of adding the fast-day horarium to excessive abstinence, to meager rations, to food preparation that was deliberately repulsive,[18] these poor monks had made the experiment with the normal vigor provided by the diet foreseen by the Rule, they would have had less trouble observing the fast. The "fevers"[19] and the other handicaps mentioned complete the explanation of their failure. St. Benedict's prescriptions cannot be held responsible for this failure, for they were applied in deplorable conditions and quite unreasonably.

From this instructive history we can draw several lessons about method, which we shall have to recall later on. For the moment, I will only underline the double conclusion drawn by Rancé: to maintain abstinence and to abandon the fasting horarium, as we see in his *Regulations.* On the one hand, he refused not only the "flesh of four-footed animals," the only food forbidden by the Benedictine Rule, but also fish, eggs and even butter.[20] On the other hand, they ate at 12:30 P.M. at the latest, with a collation in the evening, instead

18. On this, see P. Le Nain, *La Vie de Dom A.-J. Le Bouthillier de Rancé,* t. 2 (Paris, 1719), p. 576: black bread mixed with straw, oily porridge, spoiled carrots, cabbage without seasoning.... This regime was in force from 1668 to 1674, that is, during the time of the two attempts at the integral Lenten fast, and was later supposed to have been mitigated, "so that the monks could eat with less disgust" (p. 577).

19. A detail absent from the account of the two Lents in Marsollier and Gervaise, but confirmed by Le Nain, who for the years 1674–1681, speaks of more than thirty religious carried off by rheumatisms and inflammations of the lungs (p. 577).

20. Milk products remained in the diet (*Règlements,* 2nd ed., 1718, p. 19–20).

of having only one meal in the middle of the afternoon or after Vespers. Aggravation on one side, mitigation on the other: such choices unbalance the regime instituted by the Rule. By accentuating one of the elements of Benedictine ascesis at the expense of another, Rancé deprived his monks of the irreplaceable experience of the true fast, and the entire church of an example that might have suggested the revival of the primitive practice right in the midst of modern times.

But it was fated that in modern monasticism abstinence would finally triumph over the fast. When Dom Augustine de Lestrange, as in the experiment of 1672–1673, added the second of these "penances" to the first, one part of the Trappist monasteries quickly returned to Rancé's regime, and it was this regime of severe abstinence coupled with the absence of the fast strictly so called, that was taken as the basis of the 1892 union.

In the middle of the century separating Lestrange from this final abandonment of the fast, it is worthwhile to observe the behavior of a monk who went to seek at La Trappe the rigorous observance of which he dreamed. In 1849 Père Jean-Baptiste Muard, founder of La Pierre-qui-vire, returned from Italy where he had discovered the Rule of St. Benedict, and passed several months at Aiguebelle, with two companions, to be initiated into its practice. The great southern monastery was one of those that remained faithful to the Lestrange reform. "The religious eat no meal before 2:30 P.M. from September 15 on, or before 4:00 P.M. during Lent."

> Jean-Baptiste Muard's novitiate was completed precisely during the Lent of 1850. The experience was harsh. One of the Father's companions thought he was going to die of it. Well before the end of Lent, most of the religious were authorized to take the *mixt* (breakfast) at 11:30 A.M., and only Père Muard, together with Dom Orsise (the abbot of Aiguebelle) arrived at Easter having integrally observed the prescribed fasts.[21]

Thus the founder of La Pierre-qui-vire relived Rancé's experiment of 1672–1673, enduring like the eighteenth-century Trappists a Benedictine Lenten fast with a more than Benedictine abstinence. Whether or not he was instructed by this experiment,[22] he himself had to legislate for his foundation. But in his *Constitutions* we see him exactly repeating what Rance had done: abandoning the fasting horarium, he only kept abstinence and increased it as much as he could.[23]

Although Père Muard desired to conform in everything to the Rule of St. Benedict and was animated with an extreme

---

21. D. Huerre, *Jean-Baptiste Muard* (La Pierre-qui-vire, 1950), p. 317.
22. In fact, it seems that his *Constitutions* had already been drawn up at Subiaco, before his going to Aiguebelle.
23. Published only after his death (1854): *Sainte-Marie de la Pierre-qui-vire, Constitutions des Bénédictins du Sacré-Coeur-de-Jésus* (Sens, 1855). See pp. 13–14 and 48–50. Charles de Foucauld, in his turn, kept the three usual meals, while stressing the Trappist abstinence, to which he added the absence of cheese and oil, but he kept milk. See *Constitutions* 32, in Frère Charles de Jésus, *Oeuvres spirituelles, Anthologie* (Paris, 1958), p. 430 (cf. p. 549).

zeal for penitence, he judged the regular fast to be "very difficult to observe in our countries, especially during the winter, because of the harshness of the season that demands a more abundant nourishment than during the summer," and also because there was a lot of preaching activity at that time, and he wished some of his religious to preach. Therefore, while he spoke of an "all-year fast," he prescribed that the chief meal always be at noon, with a collation in the evening, the latter "quite substantial." And to compensate for this mitigation, he added to the Trappist abstinences (meat, wine, fish, eggs, butter, sugar, honey) a list of supplementary retrenchments: no cheese, no milk products, no oil. Making this abstinence "the characteristic sign of the society," he thought of binding the members of the society to it by a "special vow to observe it at all times and all places, except for cases when the Superior believes he should dispense from it."

Rancé's option appears here perfectly explicit and deliberate: in favor of abstinence and against the fast. Our nineteenth-century penitents, like those of the eighteenth century, were prepared to put up with the most meager fare, but not to forego the usual hours for eating. They imposed on themselves heroic restrictions, provided that they continued to sit down at table at noon and in the evening, like everyone else.

The appearance of breakfast

The last step in the degradation of the fast has been the establishment of breakfast. This supplementary meal, eaten at the beginning of the day, has appeared only recently. The Rule of St. Benedict and all the customaries that depend on it, speak indeed of a "piece of bread and a cup to drink" taken by the table servants on fast days before the hour of the meal, and of a *mixt* (wine mixed with water) granted to the refectory reader before he begins to read.[24] But the purpose of these anticipations was only to relieve the brothers in question from serving while fasting, seeing they will eat after the common meal, at the second table. Moreover, they only take something just before the meal, not at the beginning of the day.[25]

Although the concession of the *mixt* (a drink and some bread) was extended to children, to the sick and to lay brothers, it had not, up to the nineteenth century, engendered a true habit of breakfasting. In 1770 the *Constitutions* of St. Maur are still silent on this subject. In taking no nourishment before the midday meal, the monks, moreover, were doing nothing exceptional. The secular custom was identical. I have often heard that my great-great-grandfather, who lived in Paris during the first three-quarters of the nineteenth century, never ate anything before 11:00 A.M., when he sat down at table for lunch. He was no ascetic, but was simply following the customs of his youth.

24. RB 35, 12 and 38, 10.

25. Or at most, one hour before, according to the usual but probably erroneous interpretation of *ante unam horam refectionis* (RB 35, 12).

It was in the course of the nineteenth century that the English breakfast spread over the continent, invading religious communities as well as lay households. In some "Declarations" on the Benedictine Rule we see it introduced shamefacedly, attached as well as possible to the anticipation foreseen for the table servants: "To all our brothers we grant a dispensation to take breakfast in the morning." In fact this modern English breakfast has nothing in common with the old *mixt* of St. Benedict.

On this point the Carthusians remain faithful to the ancient custom. If their lay brothers can take a breakfast if they want, the fathers never do so. Today their pattern is no doubt unique. Breakfast has imposed itself everywhere, and the monks have docilely followed the present-day tendency to reinforce it. During my first years of religious life we ate it standing, on the run as it were. In the 1960s people thought it good to sit down at table as for the other two meals. At the same time new kinds of food were added to the original bread and coffee.

In spite of this development, breakfast has kept a sort of furtive air, which recalls its recent origin and doubtful legitimacy. No common prayer precedes it or follows it; no reading accompanies it; no set hour makes it a regular act.

Even limited by the laws of the Church and monastic regulations in penitential seasons, breakfast has completed the ruin of the fast. The name may still be used but the reality has disappeared. The midday meal with its two satellites in the morning and evening, is absolutely opposed to the one evening meal of the ancient church. As far as the monks are concerned, it must be admitted, they have not been able to maintain the ancient discipline. The conformism with which they have yielded sooner or later to the general tendency is one of the clearest signs of the deep weakness of Western monasticism in the modern period.

A Glance at the Separated Brethren

This survey of the evolution of the fast within Catholicism cannot overlook the Christian milieus around it. By contagion or by reaction they have been able to influence its behavior, and their own evolution throws light on its evolution. The harsh criticism of the Reformers, in particular, no doubt contributed to discredit the fast in the eyes of some, while arousing in others a defense and increased emphasis upon it.

The views of Luther

Fasting is often mentioned in the treatise "Good Works" of Martin Luther (1520). Usually it is only mentioned in passing in lists of works where it appears in company with prayers, alms, pilgrimages, the founding of churches, the celebration of feasts, etc. "All that," proclaims Luther, "has value only by faith; by themselves such works are worth nothing, being in no way meritorious in themselves, as people imagine."[26]

Within this general criticism of "good works," some pages treat fasting more particularly. They do so with regard to the third commandment. In his review of the Ten Commandments, Luther considers the Sabbath rest as a spiritual duty, consisting of giving oneself interior rest and leisure by mortification of the passions. The first of these "exercises of the flesh" that procures this mortification is fasting, accompanied by watching and by work. The unique aim of the fast is to appease concupiscence, and it should be regulated in view of this interior aim, without regard for external norms of frequency and duration, abstinence from particular foods, and the observance of particular days. No authority, such as that of a religious order or the Church, can dictate from without the necessary and sufficient measure which each one must fix for himself according to his needs and conscience.[27]

The double error in perspective from which Luther wants to free fasting is its being a work meritorious in itself, and an obligation imposed by authority. The practice itself does not arouse his reproof, although he seems more uneasy about those who fast too much than about those who do not fast enough.[28] What chiefly grips him is to subordinate

26. Martin Luther, *Oeuvres,* 11 (Geneva, 1957), pp. 214, 217, 220, 230.

27. Ibid., pp. 259–261. Cf. p. 272 (about the respect due to the Church) and pp. 285–287 (about chastity).

28. These latter only receive a warning at the end (p. 261).

the fast to its true end, which, according to him, is solely the mastery of the passions.

That this proposition of the Reformer was legitimate and healthy, we can easily see by his allusions to various abuses marring contemporary Christian practice: wholly exterior fasts, accompanied by compensating dainties and excessive drinking; immoderate fatigue, ruinous for the health and muddling the mind; a superstitious importance attached to certain days and certain abstinences. However, we can ask whether his criticism itself suffers from two grave defects.

The first is the strange restriction of the purpose of the fast. To make it only a means to dominate concupiscence is indeed to retain one of its major effects, but it is also to set aside many aspects that are not negligible. It is astonishing that a man so smitten by the Bible should have fallen into such a simplification. It suffices to peruse the sacred text to encounter many other meanings of the fast: mourning, penitence, "humiliation of one's soul," supplication, preparation to meet God, a sign of consecration to his service and accompaniment of a life of chastity, a weapon against the demons. The fast is all that and much more besides. No closed list of these many meanings can be established. Like every observance—and we shall return to this point—the fast is the source of innumerable meanings that reveal themselves day by day as we progress in the practice.

Besides missing these many meanings, both natural and revealed, by his reductive definition, Luther's criticism has the inconvenience of abandoning the Christian to himself, with no other guide than the vacillating light of his conscience. Luther is right to affirm that conscience can and should intervene decisively in the determination of the work to be done; but can we leave each man to his own mere good will, refraining from enacting any norm capable of enlightening and supporting that will? Scripture itself offers many examples of collective fasts "proclaimed" by authority for the welfare of all. Apart from particular circumstances when these occasional fasts take place, is it not useful, indeed necessary, for each one to be incited to fast regularly, in the framework of a community effort that moves him and gives him courage?

In a passage that would have been worthwhile to develop, Luther himself momentarily glimpsed this benefit of an education in fasting procured by the religious or ecclesial society. He expounded, regarding the sixth commandment, his purely subjective conception of the regulation of fasting, saying: "To observe oneself, to grasp what, and in what measure and for how long, will favor chastity in oneself, in order to choose it for oneself and to hold on to it." Then he added this significant phrase:

> If (the Christian) is incapable of it, let him submit himself for a time to the government of another who constrains him to it, until he becomes able to govern himself. That is why convents were

> formerly founded, to teach young people discipline and purity.[29]

In fact, that is the benefit for which I am personally indebted to the monastic tradition that guides me: it has taught me to fast. But I wonder whether it is only a passing benefit, good for beginners unable to govern themselves. Does not every Christian and every religious have permanent need of a rule that arouses, directs and supports their efforts, as a stake directs and upholds the plant?

The history of Protestantism seems to have answered that question. The disappearance of external norms enacted by authority, has led to the disappearance of the fast itself. Alas, today we can say the same of Catholicism. The absence of any serious set of laws calling Christians to fast is not one of the least deficiencies of the post-conciliar church amid the rediscovery of so many riches.

Calvin's synthesis

In passing from Luther to Calvin we find ourselves faced with much broader and reflective thought. The *Institutes of the Christian Religion* is not, like the treatise "Good Works" that we have just scanned, a rapid essay with simplistic views, but a great effort of synthesis in which fasting, like everything else, receives a serious place and deep consideration.

29. Ibid., p. 286.

Between the pure and simple rejection by certain extremist Reformers and the "superstitions" of Catholicism, Calvin traces a middle way, which attributes an important role to fasting, while purifying it of certain abuses.[30] Three ends are acknowledged for fasting. To that of "taming the flesh," with which Luther was satisfied, are added the two following: "to dispose us to prayer" and "to bear witness to our humility before God." A large selection of scriptural texts illustrates these functions; that of helping prayer receives more emphasis.

Carefully distinguishing fasting properly so-called from the simple temperance that the Christian should always observe, Calvin sets forth its modalities in detail. For him, fasting is not only a matter of time, but also of the quality of the food (which should be simple, usual, common) and of measure (to eat less and more lightly). But his principal concern is to make fasting spiritually profitable by removing several errors: hypocritical exteriority, whereas fasting is useful only as a help to inner sentiments; the illusion that sees in fasting a meritorious work in the divine service, putting this act, indifferent in itself, on the same level as the things commanded by God and necessary in themselves; the character of tyrannical obligation and sovereign importance attributed to it by a certain tradition that goes back to the Fathers of the Church themselves.

30. John Calvin, *Institution de la religion chrétienne*, Livre IV, ed. J.-D. Benoît (Paris, 1961), pp. 250–257 (chap. 12, 14–21).

This last criticism, directed against popery, was aimed especially at Lent. Calvin rejected its claim to be modelled on the Gospel—in fact, Christ did not fast to give us an example to follow—and he severely criticized its bad results. On the whole, the accent is more on relativizing the fast than on its value. While praising it theoretically, Calvin does not seem to have had in mind any well-defined practice. If he happens to recommend fasting in certain circumstances, such as public calamities, collective faults, ordinations of the ministers of the Church,[31] the verbs in the conditional tense let the reader understand that these were simple possibilities or wishes, if you will, inspired by scripture but not corresponding to any lived reality. The tendency is the same as with Luther, echoes of whom are recognizable here and there. The tendency is towards the disappearance of fasting, first as an ecclesial observance, but consequently also as a private practice.

In this regard we can ask if the correction of existing abuses has not been a remedy that is worse than the sickness. Péguy's words recur to me: "Kantianism has pure hands, but it has no hands." Whether or not these words are fair to the German philosopher, they could be repeated in regard to the Church and fasting. Desiring to purify fasting, we have killed it. Were not all its defects in the end less grave than the total effacement of it, which is our present state?

31. Livre III, p. 83–84 (chap. 3, 17) and 109 (chap. 4, 11); Livre IV, p. 66 (chap. 3, 12).

Anglicanism: Pusey and Newman

This impression produced by the criticism of the great Reformers is confirmed by the considerations developed two centuries later by the promoters of the Oxford Movement. In a tract dated December 21, 1833, Pusey pleaded lengthily in favor of resuming the "system of fasts prescribed by our Church."[32] Anglicanism indeed has preserved an impressive calendar that recalls its Catholic origins: no less than one hundred and eight days, or two-sevenths of the year, are fast days. But the complaints and remonstrances of the author of the tract show that this fine program became a dead letter: "Our Church," he notes, "has left to Christian prudence and each one's experience the care of determining *how* he should fast."[33] Although, as a respectful son of the church, Pusey does not criticize this liberty left to its members, clearly the absence of precise directives has resulted in the collapse of the practice, which in the first third of the nineteenth century was at the point of death.

With admirable intelligence and courage, visibly inspired by personal experience of what he is promoting, Pusey tries to reanimate the old dying discipline. His pleading is excellent, but the reader guesses he will scarcely be heard. A postscript avows that this appeal to ecclesiastical discipline runs

32. *Tract 18: Thoughts on the Benefits of the System of Fasting Enjoined by our Church.* I cite the London 1845 edition. See p. 10, the enumeration of the fast days.

33. Ibid., p. 7.

into an objection: are not the laws of the Church in this matter virtually abrogated by long desuetude? Everything acts as if "the Church herself had tacitly abandoned them."[34] This remark shows that the abandonment is of long standing, and suggests that Anglicanism had sunk several centuries earlier into the impotence we know.

A few days after this *Tract 18*, Newman launched another one, anonymous and much shorter, entitled "Mortification of the Flesh: a Duty According to Scripture."[35] Moses, Elijah and Daniel, John the Baptist, the Apostles and the Fathers are cited as examples of the practice of fasting in the two Testaments and in the ancient church, by a man who also knew what he was talking about. But the argumentation shows the depth of the evil. The "people" whom Newman addressed were in no ways persuaded that fasting and the other exercises of mortification had their place in Christian life. The author recognized that at present "what is in reality self-indulgence passes for a simple, moderate and innocent use of the goods of this world."

Contemporary Orthodoxy

This glance at our separated brothers obviously cannot neglect the Orthodox Churches. Having seen already that at a very early date they renounced the principle of the single

34. Ibid., p. 26.
35. *Tract 21* (January 1, 1834).

meal, we are not surprised to find today that their "fast" is compatible with several meals. Only breakfast is in principle prohibited during Lent, the fast being therefore total until noon.[36] On the other hand, the abstinence is rigorous: not only meat, but also milk foods and eggs, even fish, are most often prohibited in certain churches. Moreover, the calendar is overloaded: to the pre-Easter Lent are added other Lents before June 29 and August 15, a long Advent of forty days, Wednesdays and Fridays of every week almost all year, and finally some vigils and feasts.

While such a program is presented to the faithful, it is important to note that the Church does not impose it as a law, but proposes it as a model, leaving each one to adapt it to his own possibilities. In fact, most observe a mitigated Lent. We are even told that many, discouraged by a model that surpasses them, do nothing at all. This quite general mitigation, reaching to a complete lack of observance, attests to a malaise that is not unlike the flabbiness of Western Christianity. However, Orthodoxy can congratulate itself on maintaining a concrete demand and arousing a real effort. This traditional and still living norm remains a base, always available for reflection, experimentation and renewal.

36. I borrow from C. Bendaly, "Jeûne et oralité. Aspects psychologiques du jeûne orthodoxe et suggestions pour une éventuelle réform," in *Contacts 37* (1985), pp. 163–219 (see p. 199–200). For the Syrian Churches, see the remarks in Régamey, *Redécouverte*, pp. 329–335.

Catholicism again: the theologians and the monks

It was the same only a short while ago in Catholicism, when the laws of the Church, in spite of all the mitigations, continued to maintain a certain consciousness of the necessity of fasting. However, it must be recognized that the meaning of its benefits was scarcely any longer perceived. When we consult the article on "Fasting" (*Jeûne*) in the great ecclesial encyclopedia, the *Dictionnaire de théologie catholique*, we are abashed to find there only a review of the Christian's obligations and loopholes in this matter.[37] Written only a half-century ago, these pages are filled only with legalism and casuistry, without the least spiritual breath. This deep poverty foretells the coming abolition of the fast even more than the innumerable twists given to the law that are mentioned there.

In the monastic world the climate was scarcely any better, if we judge by modern commentaries on the Rule. Paradoxically, they join generous praise for Benedictine "discretion" with complete silence on the non-observance of Benedict's prescriptions. On the one hand, they praise the Father of monks for having admirably tempered the traditional austerities so that little or nothing of them remains. On the other hand, they do not even mention that his meal program, reputed to be so easy, is in fact completely ignored.

37. A. Thouvenin, "Carême," *DTC* 8 (1925), col. 1411–1417.

But if the Rule is so generous and human, why do the monks keep from practicing it, as if it demanded frightful austerities? In reality, the revulsion inspired by fasting explains both the celebration of Benedict's discretion and the silence on the application of his norms. By praising Benedict for having mitigated the observances of his predecessors, the monks absolve themselves implicitly for not being faithful to his.

What has Killed Fasting?

This survey of the Christian world has thus brought us face to face with a universal problem. No church, no religious society, seems exempt from serious difficulties, if not total allergy, relative to this great biblical act of fasting, which is part of our common patrimony. The disaffection for it is particularly astonishing among the monks, who originally were devoted to cultivating it with predilection.

Thus we are brought back to our initial question: why this death of fasting even where it should be especially alive? At present we know a little better how the monks arrived at this point, together with the Christian people, whose evolution they have but followed. Since it is a general phenomenon, we must seek an explanation on the level of the whole church. As I have said, the real motive cannot be the physical enfeeblement of the human system, nor work, nor social life. What is it then?

"The flesh is weak"

First of all, we must certainly take into account a "weakness of the flesh" (I do not say weakness of health), which pertains to all ages. Because fasting is inconvenient and demands effort, it is bound to deteriorate at the least weakening of wills. "The spirit is willing" to start fasting, but "the flesh is weak" in maintaining it.

The maintenance of such a practice supposes an ever alert attention and a constant renewal of generosity. If preaching does not regularly breathe into it adequate motivation, it soon dries up and disappears. Christian fasting has disappeared, because pastors and faithful have not reinvented it together in each generation.

A disincarnate spirituality

Besides this general cause, more specific sicknesses have doubtless attacked fasting. One of them seems to be a certain modern spiritualism, which tends to disdain bodily works and to be interested only in states of soul. When ideas and sentiments are the only things that count, a practice as material as fasting cuts a paltry figure.

Pusey noted this fact already: for many of his readers, "to renounce oneself in such a lowly matter as food is something so shabby and insignificant that the doctrine of the Cross would be degraded by founding on it such an observance."[38]

38. *Tract 18*, pp. 21–22.

To which Pusey justly replies that little actions repeated make the great habits that characterize the person. Moreover, "the motive ennobles the action, the action does not dishonor the motive." Religion is not being degraded by being engaged in practices of this sort, but confers on fasting a religious dimension that completes and sanctifies it.

Even if I must be reckoned a materialist, I shall add that I scarcely believe in a spirituality that is content with interior states. Just as it is unhealthy to be content with observances without caring about what goes on inside, so we are deceived by cultivating sentiments not translated into any practice. Pharisaic exteriority has a no less deadly counterpart: pure inferiority, combining beautiful states of soul with middle-class comfort. True spirituality is one that is incarnate in acts. The realism of the ancients understood this well. To despise these concrete practices that make the man is to separate the soul from the body, to enter into a sort of death, to fall into angelism and illusion.

This great modern illusion has deep roots. As early as the twelfth century we see it outlined in the correspondence of an exceptionally intelligent and cultivated person, Heloise, the friend of Abelard. As a nun and superior, she asked her former lover, who had become her spiritual director, to compose a rule for her and her sisters. Among her requests, the one she develops at greatest length has to do with a question of food.[39]

39. Heloise, *Ep.* 6 (5 Muckle), *PL* 178:213–226 (see 218–225).

No doubt it deals less with fasting than with abstinence—Heloise wanted them to be authorized to eat meat—but a good part of the arguments are so general that all food discipline, indeed all exterior observance, is shaken by them.

Since women are weaker than men (!) and the monks themselves now show they are unable to practice the ancient rigors, the Abbess of the Paraclete would therefore like the nuns dispensed for good from abstaining from meat and from other outdated renunciations. Sin is the only thing that God commands us to avoid. But to eat meat is not a sin. Let us not count exterior actions as important as the Jews do, for they do not make us more pleasing to God. The only thing that matters is the interior that distinguishes us from the Jews, and the charity that distinguishes us from the wicked. Then follows an abundant display of New Testament texts in which are especially paraded everything said by St. Paul discrediting the dietary observances of Jewish and Gnostic inspiration.

But Heloise was not content to cite these scriptural texts already invoked in the fourth century by the adversaries of asceticism, whom Saint Jerome cut to pieces. She also reproduces a series of extracts from Saint Augustine, and thinks she can draw from this holy doctor such propositions as these:

> Exterior works add nothing to merit.... Only the virtues are meritorious before God.... The whole

> business of true Christians is to adorn the inner man with virtues and to cleanse him of vices; they have no care, or almost no care, for the exterior.[40]

Fasting therefore, together with everything external and visible, has little importance for this disciple of Augustine, who would doubtless have astonished her master.

Abelard in his reply echoes these considerations, while adding many others of his own.[41] That these Christian intellectuals of the twelfth century, the flower of the university milieu from which would arise the modern intelligentsia, should regard bodily ascesis with such disdain, is a harbinger of the evil from which we suffer. One of their favorite themes, inherited from ancient philosophy, was the appeal to "nature" and "necessity." Very good, but what does that tell us? The whole problem is precisely to discern true human necessity from the necessity imposed by habits and prejudices. To establish the latter as a law is to install oneself in a comfortable mediocrity and to prohibit all fruitful effort.

A penal conception of fasting

Another evil has visibly eroded the observance of fasting: the juridical spirit that sees in it only a way of making reparation for sin. This penal conception of fasting has not only caused

40. Ibid., 222–223, citations from Augustine, *De bono coniugali* 25–27.
41. Abelard, *Ep.* 8 (7 McLaughlin), PL 178:255–314 (see 267–280, especially 275–276).

it to seem sad and unattractive, but it also engenders the idea that it can be commuted to other equivalent punishments. The intrinsic and irreplaceable value of fasting thus disappears from sight: it is only one way among others to afflict oneself.

By the way in which theologians and pastors often use the principle of compensation in this field, we see that this aspect of a punishment to be worked off has in the end dominated the ecclesiastical mentality. Even the excellent *Traité des jeûnes* by Thomassin (1680) has only this conclusion: since the Church's ancient discipline is so weakened, the Christian should compensate for this deficit of penitence by an extra amount of prayers and good works.[42]

In one monastic congregation of the same era, there was also the wish to "compensate" for the numerous derogations from the Rule in the matter of fasting by "other abstinences." Therefore it was decreed that the monks would fast (with a mitigated "fast" of course) every Friday, even during Easter time.[43] In this case the compensation had the merit of staying within the domain of food, but the failure was only made more clear: by adding some Fridays to the calendar of

42. L. Thomassin, *Traité*, pp. 562–565. Already in the sixth century Caesarius of Arles, *Serm.* 199, 1, wanted the faithful who could not fast to compensate by giving more in alms. But this was only the corollary of a conception of fasting that combined it with charity: when one of them was impossible, the other remained open.

43. *Regula S. Benedicti...cum Declarationibus...Congregationis Casinensis* (Venice, 1723), p. 89. This perpetual Friday fast, which reminds us of the Carthusians, is also found at Saint Maur (Constitutions of 1770, p. 131).

the Rule has the degradation of the whole observance been redeemed?

Similarly in the middle of the nineteenth century, Père Muard intended to compensate for the mitigation of the fast by the very strict abstinence of which I have spoken. This time the compensation was certainly heavy enough to procure a genuine penitential equivalence on the level of affliction, but it did not restore the specific effects and benefits of fasting any more than any other substitute would.

The system of compensation has thus reigned in the Church, replacing fasting with substitutes that the qualified authorities were proficient in weighing. Justice was saved, as well as mercy: the Lord had his due, and sin its chastisement. But however vigilant this control of the changes was, it lost the essential: the richness of the meaning and the multiform virtue of fasting, reduced to the unpleasant role of punishment.

This impoverished notion of fasting has doubtless done more harm than anything else, first of all, obviously, by stirring people to replace it with other punishments that are reputed to be equally hard. But also because it makes fasting appear as one of those "odious" things which a canonical principle wishes to be "restricted" as far as possible.[44] From

44. *Odiosa sunt restringenda*, a principle which Dom A. Calmet, *Commentaire littéral, historique et moral sur la Règle de saint Benoît*, t. 2 (Paris, 1734), p. 47, paraphrases thus: "In regard to laws and regulations, prohibitions, as being odious, should be restricted, and limited to the precise terms of the law or the prohibition."

that root springs the general connivance on the part of legislators and subjects of the law, constantly to blunt the obligation of the discipline and its bite.

The constant tendency to reduction, so striking in the course of these centuries of inexorable decline, is not explained solely by negligence or cowardice. It proceeds from more profoundly from a crisis of thought. The fast has died from the narrow concept in which it was enclosed. Conceived as a punishment, or at best as a sacrifice, it was particularly exposed to danger in an age when the sense of sin was going to grow feeble, in which the fear of God's justice would yield more and more to a quasi-exclusive accent on his goodness.

Is fasting replaced by obedience?

Western monasticism has not been able to enlarge this skimpy concept of fasting to the dimensions of its own traditional doctrine. I have just cited two cases of monastic milieus that claimed to "compensate" with other austerities for the abandonment of the fast, as was done in contemporary ecclesiastical society. However, there is another way, much more radical, of getting rid not only of fasting but of all corporal austerity. It is to make the common life, and especially obedience, a substitute for these exterior "penitences."

The theory of this substitution was elaborated by Dom Cuthbert Butler, who attributed it to St. Benedict himself. According to this English Benedictine at the beginning of this century, Benedict would have broken with the previous tradition of monasticism, which put the accent on austerities, to direct the religious life towards another ideal: the integral common life, obedience being the supreme renunciation, because it was spiritual.[45]

To believe that Benedict eliminated corporal austerity from monastic life is an error, as I have said, and it is proved by our own repugnance to follow him. The Rule indeed insists on the common life and on the interior mortification of obedience. But this insistence, which is nothing peculiar to it at all,[46] does not mean that the other elements of monastic ascesis are without importance. However precious these communitarian values, however lofty obedience, the personal ascesis of fasting and analogous bodily practices remain irreplaceable, being of another order.

Conclusion

Butler's thesis has deeply penetrated the monasteries, since it corresponds to the present-day Benedictine practice and justifies it. This capitulation is the last stage on the decline. When we come to legitimize the decline, and what is more, to see it as progress, no reason exists to reform ourselves. Every effort in this direction even becomes suspect.

45. C. Butler, *Benedictine Monachism* (London, 1924), pp. 21–26 (chap. 2, end–chap. 3, section 1) and 45 (end of chap. 4); see also pp. 300–301 (chap. 8, middle).

46. One example among many: Gregory the Great, *Commentary on Kings* II, 127 and VI, 29–32, declares obedience superior to all austerities, but he also notes that the latter are indispensable.

Not only does contemporary monastic life not inspire people to fast, but it prevents them. Both in Europe and in America I have met young people who used to fast before becoming monks, but as soon as they entered the monastery, there could be no question of it. This phenomenon is astonishing for whoever knows the slightest bit of the origins and tradition of monasticism, and merits the most serious attention. I shall say no more about it, for I must reflect on a complementary subject: the means of climbing back up this slope and finding again the lost fast.

CHAPTER V

Toward a Resurrection: To Love Fasting

THE LAST words of the title just above are not mine. I take them from the Rule of St. Benedict. In the list of "The Tools for Good Works" that comprises a whole chapter, the Rule contains this sentence: *Jejunium amare.*[1] I have already noted the significant position of this appeal for fasting: after the Pauline maxim "punish your body," and before the evangelical precept "relieve the lot of the poor" (see Chapter III, note 29). Fasting as a fundamental practice of Christian asceticism blossoms into generosity towards one's neighbor. But at present it is the very content of the sentence "To love fasting" that holds my attention. Is it possible? Let us admit that the combination of the two words sounds paradoxical. If there is one thing we don't love spontaneously, it is fasting!

A condition sine qua non

And yet we must indeed love fasting if we wish it to be alive and practiced. The preceding chapter has shown well enough that when considered a mere affliction, something odious, fasting perishes: *Odiosa sunt restringenda.* Just as we inevitably

1. Benedict (RB 4:13) here reproduces the Master (RM 3:13).

tend to reduce and suppress what we do not love, so we keep and develop what we love. St. Benedict's saying gives the pertinent and providential reply to the canonical principle just mentioned ("Odious things are to be restricted"). The Rule is right: "to love fasting" is the only way to revive it.

Love is inventive and enterprising. If we love fasting, the game is won. Obstacles will not be lacking, but none of them will block us. The whole problem engaging us is therefore reduced to the combination of this verb and this noun. Its being a paradox does not prevent its being true. To love fasting is not only possible. In the light of the facts, I will go so far as to say that the contrary appears impossible to me, to whatever degree one has truly experienced fasting. Experience fasting, and you will love it.

The benefits of the fast speak for themselves. It is enough to experience them. But how to obtain this experience? A person does not impose such an effort on himself without being moved by an attraction that is already a kind of love. Thus a vicious circle is established. To love fasting one must experience it, but to experience it, one must love it. The way to get out of this circle is easy: trust in the word of God, in the example of the saints, in the great voice of tradition, and trusting in this witness, try it. That is how I myself began. And as much as I remain a beginner, I wish to add my tiny witness as a modern man to the centuries-old dossier.

The present situation

Although ultimately each person and each community must make a leap in the dark, incentives and reassurances are close at hand. At present, many elements favor a return to fasting. Among them we must first mention the renewed sense of the role of the body in the spiritual life. The title of the collection *Wisdom of the Body* says much about the contemporary rediscovery of man as a unity of flesh and spirit. We can no longer be content with fine sentiments and good works.

Between an interior life that ignores the body and exterior action that employs it as a mere tool, we need an incarnate spirituality that makes grace descend into our whole being.

This demand is not only felt by many Christians at the grassroots level, but is also affirmed in statements from one of the highest authorities of the Church, declaring it necessary to "find again the bodily aspect even of faith." Speaking of fasting, the same voice insists that the sense of personal responsibility, emphasized by the liberty left to each one in the past few decades, be combined with "common expressions of ecclesial penitence," that is urgent to recover.[2] The present void is thus perceived as an appeal to create something. In this effort to restore penitential observances to the

2. J. Ratzinger, V. Messori, *The Ratzinger Report* (San Francisco: Ignatius Press, 1985), pp. 113–114. The Second Vatican Council, in the only passage in which it refers to the Christian fast (*Nostra etate*, the Declaration on Non-Christian Religions, praises that of Islam), said that "during Lent, penance should not be only internal and individual but also external and social" (*Sacrosanctum Concilium*, 110).

whole church, do not the monks have the capacity as well as the duty to make an exemplary contribution, drawn from the treasury of their own tradition?

Their negligence in this regard is more regrettable since the recent revival of some practice of fasting among Christians. The above passage from Cardinal Ratzinger was provoked by the events of Medjugorje. One of the most striking results of these apparitions has been to restore to honor the ancient fasts on Fridays and even Wednesdays. Old Christian habits going back to the time of the spread of Islam[3] have thus returned to vigor in this corner of Herzegovina and are spreading with surprising rapidity.[4]

To these movements taking shape in the very bosom of Catholicism are to be added other parallels, whether religious or not, which we met earlier in the review of ancient and modern practices. In contemporary civilization, fasting has become a current, sometimes spectacular, instrument of political protest. Quietly, it serves to express and sustain solidarity with a Third World that is undernourished or even starving. Medically, it is used to treat overfed Westerners. Finally, several spiritual traditions, such as Greek Orthodoxy, Islam and Hinduism, keep it alive before our eyes at a time when journeys and intercultural contacts are more numerous.

3. On this historical background, see H. Joyeux, R. Laurentin, *Etudes médicales et scientifiques sur les apparitions de Medjugorje* (Paris, 1985), p. 99–100.

4. See, among others, S. Barbarie, *Le Pain des pauvres. Invitation aux chrétiens à jeûner* (Hauteville: Ed. du Parvis, 1985).

For a specifically monastic fast

These many appeals are well suited to help monasticism find its lost observance, and some of them, especially those related to the Third World, have already aroused some response. But the stimulation brought by them has its dangers. By presenting ready-made models with their particular modes and motivations, they risk introducing foreign elements into monastic life that cannot be harmoniously integrated. Thus it is very important that monks turn to their own tradition to draw forms of fasting homogeneous with their life and adapted to their program.

Evidently the Rule of St. Benedict can and should render us the greatest help in this search for a practice of fasting that is not an artificial borrowing from without, but a growth from within the monastic life. In the Rule we have a dietary regime that was conceived for monks as part of their way of life. In following it, we shall not deviate from our vocation, but shall restore a fundamental element of it that has been strangely abandoned for generations.

In the wake of Vatican II

Without excluding recourse to other monastic sources, it seems that the first step towards a rediscovery of fasting in monasteries should therefore be a movement to come closer to the Rule.

When Vatican II invited religious "to set in full light and to safeguard faithfully the spirit of the founders and their specific intentions, as well as their wholesome traditions" did it not imply an effort in this direction?[5] If there is one great and healthy monastic tradition, carefully regulated by the Father of monks, it is indeed the tradition of fasting. The fact that it has been interrupted and consequently cannot be "maintained" but must be recreated only adds to the urgency. Or are monks and other religious condemned only to preserve what has come down to them, without reviving what has wrongfully perished?

The objection will no doubt be made that adaptation to the present is another of the Council's prescriptions, and that this is absolutely opposed to a return to the fast as it was practiced fifteen centuries ago. Is not St. Benedict's regime, like many other things in the Rule, tied to an age and civilization far removed from ours? Does not its progressive abandonment during the centuries prove that it is impossible for modern man? The regular fast may be one of those "obsolete" things which Vatican II, far from encouraging us to restore, bids us on the contrary to "suppress" even in its last traces.[6]

The monastic fast and secular habits yesterday and today

These objections are worth considering. The objection that ties fasting to the customs of antiquity is sometimes

5. *Perfectae caritatis*, 2.
6. Ibid., 3.

supported by considerations of the climate. It is said that Mediterranean man is not used to eating early in the morning or is content with very little at that hour.[7] But North European man needs to eat more to resist the cold. Thus the Anglo-Saxon breakfast, which is so widespread in recent times, is justified. Anyway, the monastic regime seems inseparable from secular habits. Ancient civilization and the Mediterranean climate shaped the meal times fixed by St. Benedict. In different times and climates, everything has to be revised according to different customs.

I do not deny the relationship between ancient monasticism and its cultural context, but I do believe that the dependence of the first on the second has been exaggerated. There is, of course, continuity between the two, but also rupture. When someone like Dom Cuthbert Butler presents the regime in the Rule as practically identical to that of the laity of the time, he misses some important differences of which I would like to give an idea.

To begin with breakfast, which St. Benedict's monks never had, its absence was not a general, automatic fact. A distinction should be made among the various levels of society. In a piece of Christian fiction that may date from the third century, the *Recognitions* of Pseudo-Clement, we find

7. Cuthbert Butler, *Benedictine Monachism*, p. 42, citing the American traveller M. Crawford. An idea repeated recently by E. de Bhaldraithe, "Monasticism in the United States," in *Religious Life Review* 25 (Dublin, 1986), p. 4–10 (see p. 8).

an interesting note on this point. The hero, who belongs to the highest social class, did not eat before the seventh hour (1:00 P.M.) while living in Rome. During a sea voyage from Italy to Palestine, he would eat at daybreak, as did the sailors on board, and once he acquired this habit he had difficulty breaking it.[8]

This anecdote gives a glimpse of two simultaneous practices: that of manual workers who ate very early before going to work, and that of other milieus where people broke their fast around noon. Let it be said in passing that this difference was probably perpetuated. When I mentioned above that my great-great-grandfather ate nothing before 11:00 A.M., I should have made clear that he was not a manual worker. On the contrary, manual workers of his time, like those of antiquity, no doubt ate early in the morning. Such, at any rate, seems to have been the habit of the peasant milieu from which Père Muard came, to judge by the sacrifice it seemed to be for him to give up breakfast.[9] Moreover, it is well known that some monastic customaries grant lay-brothers

8. Clement, *Recognitiones* II, 2, 3–4. Although breakfast was usual for the sailors of the third century A.D., according to Pseudo-Clement, it does not seem to have been the custom for soldiers five centuries earlier. See Titus Livius, *Hist.* 21, 54–55: the victory of the Carthaginians over the Romans at Trebia in very cold weather was due largely to the fact that Hannibal had ordered the Carthaginians to eat breakfast at dawn, while the Romans remained fasting.

9. Abbé Brullée, *Vie du R. P. Muard* (Sens, 1863), p. 266. However, the morning breakfast that J. B. Muard renounces might have been a habit acquired in the seminary.

and laymen doing heavy work a *mixt* that is not granted to the monks who are clerics.[10]

To return to the time of St. Benedict, the story of Pseudo-Clement suggests that the peasants around Monte Cassino, like other field workers, ate breakfast before going to the fields. Was it less abundant than the English breakfast of the twentieth century? It is possible, but its absence must have been felt keenly by the monks, who did manual labor for several hours starting at daybreak. This privation was increased by the fact that they rose very early. Rising at two or three o'clock in the morning, they fasted much longer than the lay people.

Regarding the *prandium* (noon meal), the ancients did not consider it as important as the *cena* (evening meal), but it was nonetheless part of a normal day. An author in fifth-century Gaul, Sidonius Apollinaris, has left us two descriptions of typical days, one of the Visigothic King Theodoric in his capital of Toulouse, and the other of the writer himself during a stay with friends near Nîmes.[11] In each case the meal is either around noon, or at the end of the fifth hour (11:00 A.M.), followed by a "meridien" or siesta. In each case the meal also qualifies as "abundant," with the addition

10. Thus Rancé granted the lay brothers six ounces of bread (about 180 grams); cf. *Réglements de l'abbaye de Notre-Dame de la Trappe* (Paris, 1718), p. 23. The same ration existed at Aiguebelle and La Pierre-qui-Vire in Père Muard's time. Today the Carthusian lay-brothers have an optioned breakfast.

11. Sidonius Apollinaris, *Letters* I, 2, 6–7; II, 9, 6.

in the first case, "in the Gallican style." A still more ample *cena* in the evening succeeds this noon meal.

Compared with this regime for lay Christians, the one meal of the monastic fast, eaten either in the middle or the end of the afternoon, seems like a severe penance. Every Wednesday and Friday in summer, and perhaps more often,[12] every weekday from September 13 to Easter, the monks did without one of the two elements of the ordinary meal schedule.

Regarding both breakfast and the noon meal, monastic practice is therefore considerably more restricted than secular custom. The latter, whatever people may say, was not very different from ours. The true chasm is not between the ancient and modern worlds, but between secular life and the ancient monastic life.

Therefore, there is no reason to claim that monastic life today should conform to contemporary secular custom. While taking account of it, monasticism should, if it wishes to be itself, vigorously detach itself from secular custom by a clearly different meal schedule. Reintroducing the regular fast is not returning to the obsolete customs of a race that has disappeared. It is to rediscover an essential trait of monasticism, regardless of the epoch to which it belongs. Today, as in the past, the monk is one who separates himself

12. It is not certain that the midday meal (*prandium*) was combined with an evening meal (*cena*) on summer days when the monks were not fasting.

from society, and this separation for the sake of God should be marked in his flesh as well as in his spirit, in his way of eating as well as in the way he regards creatures and the Creator.

Does the monk cease to belong to his own time if he does not conform to the common schedule for meals? Allow me to raise a doubt. St. Benedict and his monks seem to us to be obviously men of the sixth century, as they were. Today's monks would not be less twentieth-century men by departing from contemporary custom as earlier monks did. In this way we could bring to our own century an interesting and useful contribution, far superior to our present conformity. Who belongs more to this century? The one who sings in unison with the majority or the one who enriches the song with an original note—one who has something to offer with a loving heart to the men of his time?

Of course this difference between monks and laymen, which we observe in the past and commend for the present, does not prevent the eating habits of both from having certain traits in common that are characteristic of their common epoch. Similarly, belonging to a particular region imposes on all, religious or not, the same particularities caused by the food available or the climate. If southerners and northerners have different needs, it is normal that these differences are felt by monks as well. Sidonius Apollinaris, as I note above, emphasizes the "abundance" of the laity's meals in Gaul. A half-century earlier, another Aquitainian writer, Sulpicius Severus, also derided the gross appetite of the monks in Gaul, compared to their confreres in Egypt.[13]

Perhaps climatic reasons of this sort partially explain certain habits originating in Anglo-Saxon countries, as we suggest above. But it would surely be an exaggeration to reduce the regime of the ancient monks and of St. Benedict to a matter of climate. In every latitude, monastic life is bound to distance itself from current custom. Circumstances of place and time change nothing in this fundamental law, which applies wherever a monasticism worthy of the name develops. The monastic regime may be affected in its concrete modes by the different regions where the monks live. But is the essential trait of the regular fast, the one daily meal taken late in the day, subject to these variations? What prevents us from practicing it today is not a matter of place, but of will.

The alleged decline in human strength

Returning to the temporal dimension, I must again reckon with the current objection of the enfeeblement of health. This is another way of eliminating fasting in the name of history. Just as some would like to connect it with a dead civilization, others, and no doubt many more, imagine that it was combined with a physical vigor which modern man lacks. They think of humanity as an ailing old lady, doomed to inevitable decline. It is a painful view, of course, but very

13. Sulpicius Severus, *Dialogues* I, 4–5; II, 8.

comforting because it dispenses from all effort. The monastic fast, they think, has had its time. It is no longer possible for the man and the monk of today.

As I have said, my modest experience has proved to me that this is an error. I have good health, but not much physical vigor or moral courage; yet I easily arrived, by small stages, at practicing and surpassing the whole program of the Rule. Knowing my limits and that I am in no sense a "tough," I am ready to assure my contemporaries that their strength as modern men is abundantly sufficient to apply the prescriptions of St. Benedict.

I shall add an important detail: neither today nor formerly does the imposition of the regime of the Rule oblige one to renounce work or even to limit it. One who submits to the regular fast is not diminished either physically, intellectually, or *a fortiori* spiritually. On the contrary, he benefits from increased vigor, chiefly in his spiritual life, but also in all the domains of his activity.

Modern man is therefore capable of fasting just as his fathers. The fasts of our contemporaries prove this superabundantly. Why then could not the modern monk do so? Why does he not do so, except that he has no good reasons to do so, or gives himself bad reasons for not doing so? The astonishing absence of fasting in modern monastic life is not the result of physical, but of psychic causes. It is not strength, but motives that are lacking. The convenient presumption of weakness that reigns today in monastic circles, does not date from yesterday. As early as the twelfth century we saw it outlined in Heloise's letter to Abelard of which we have spoken. Especially in regard to the nuns but also to the monks, the abbess of the Paraclete did not believe in the possibility of maintaining the ascetic discipline of the Fathers in her time. This intellectual woman, laboring under doubts concerning the Christian meaning of such ascesis, invokes the natural weakness of women and the habits of contemporary men to declare the discipline impossible.

One hundred years later Saint Clare and her sisters refuted by their deeds this supposed impossibility. Not only was abstinence from meat, which Heloise judged inhuman, observed by them as an inviolable rule, but they imposed on themselves in perpetuity to take only Lenten fare on feast days and ferial days alike, and moreover to fast every day except Sundays and Christmas Day.[14]

This contrast between the Paraclete and Assisi, a century apart, illumines the true nature of the options for or against ascesis. According to the views of Heloise and the myth of decline familiar to us, the judgment of weakness in the twelfth century could only be confirmed in the thirteenth. But the rising of spiritual sap in the thirteenth century brought about the flourishing of renewed practices that

14. Clare of Assisi, "Third Letter to Agnes of Prague" (1328), 29–37; *Rule* 3, 8–11, in *Ecrits* (Paris, 1985), SC 325, pp. 106–108 and 130–132. In the first document, fasting is optional on Thursdays, and dispensed with in Paschal time, as well as on feasts of the Virgin and of the Apostles.

seemed to belong to a different age. And this among the women, whose weakness Heloise constantly emphasized.[15] Nothing better demonstrates that the regular fast is always possible to one who wants it, and is impossible only to one who does not want it.

Fasting is certainly possible, even easy, today, for one like myself, who is free to organize his life and to establish his time schedule as he likes. For a community, it is obviously much less easy, but not impossible. The number and diversity of persons, the delicate health of some and everyone's habits, relations with the world and the necessities of particular tasks, all that sets up a series of considerable obstacles to a renewal in the matter of fasting. If we add that the average age in many monasteries as well as in the general European population, is often elevated these last years, everything can seem to militate for the maintenance of the status quo.

Yet these forces of inertia are in danger of being overthrown by the evidence springing forth both from ancient texts and contemporary witness: fasting is beneficial, possible, necessary. The Council's appeal for renewal has not lost its edge; the *aggiornamento* of monastic life is not finished. The *renovatio accommodata* of Vatican II, considered under

15. The first Franciscans had a more generous regime, in which, however, fasting had a notable place. See *Regula* I, 3,11–13 (cf. 9, 11–16): fasting from All Saints to Christmas, from Epiphany to Easter and all Fridays, but no abstinence; II, 3, 5–14: fasting becomes optional from Epiphany to Lent, dispensation from abstinence is limited to journeys. Cf. Francis of Assisi, *Ecrits* (Paris, 1981), SC 285, pp. 128 (cf. p. 142) and 186.

its two aspects of return to the sources and adaptation to the present time, seems to demand an inventive effort in this direction. To establish a connection again with this great tradition of fasting no doubt would constitute a more serious and substantial *aggiornamento* than the haphazard modernization of merely customary habits.

The meanings of fasting

Since we only lack convictions and motives, it is not idle to review those pointed out in the preceding pages. Fasting is not only the mastery of desire on a key point, commanding the whole complex of human appetites. It is also the repose of the digestive functions, the cessation of the violence done to living things destroyed by these functions, the recollection of man within himself in a sort of detachment and self-sufficiency. From these spring pacification and spiritual refinement obtained, both when the fasting period is finished, and in the whole way of life in which fasting recurs at regular intervals.

While fasting by its nature purifies soul and body, in addition it is for the Christian a combat in company with Christ in the desert, the commemoration of the Bridegroom's departure, and waiting for his return. For the monk it is the companion of chastity, the brother of solitude and silence, the associate of prayer, the ally of meditation nourishing itself on the word of God.

The primacy of practice

I could continue this litany, but shall refrain. Continuing would suggest that I mean to give a complete catalogue of the properties and meanings of the fast. But I want to suggest just the contrary. To my way of thinking, the list remains wide open, and should so remain.

Ascetic practices and observances resemble written texts. In the latter, structuralism teaches us to see inexhaustible and ever-active sources of meaning. For each reader and for each act of reading, the text gives forth a particular message, with tones and nuances that are always new.

It is the same for fasting. Practice it and it will be a source of many meanings, unforeseeable and undefined. Tradition, by its multiform interpretations, already lets us foresee this limitless richness. Experience in its turn will show that it is impossible to contain in a closed list the meanings that the fast takes on, day by day, for those who live it.

That is why it is more important to practice fasting than to define it. The Cartesian approach that demands a clear and distinct idea of the purposes aimed at, is opposed by the traditional pedagogy of monasticism, which prefers that the monk discover the meaning of things by doing them. One of Cassian's old men puts it admirably: "The knowledge of all things will follow through experience of the work."[16]

---

16. Cassian, *Conferences* 18, 3, 1: "Per operis experientiam etiam rerum omnium scientia subsequetur."

Therefore I have no pretension of establishing *a priori* what ends fasting will serve, or how one arrives at that result. The motivations I sketch are only appeals to an experiment that each one should make for himself, and which will reveal *every* thing to him day by day.

Let us remember Luther and his simplistic limitation of the purposes of fasting. That is the opposite of what we should do, which is to leave to fasting its spread of indefinitely varied meanings. The concrete forms it has taken and takes every day, are numberless, as we have seen. Innumerable *a fortiori* are the meanings that these distinct practices take on, in proportion as each faster carries them out in each circumstance.

Fasting: easy or difficult?

Therefore we should enter upon the traditional practice of fasting with a minimum of preconceived ideas. The Rule for monks calls us to it; the monastic life invites us to it by its whole orientation and dynamism. This internal logic of our vocation, combined with the example of the Fathers, should be capable of moving us. To set us to work, it suffices us to believe, on the witness of tradition, that fasting is beneficial and possible, without knowing exactly how.

Earlier, I said it was possible and even easy. Perhaps this was imprudent. To speak of easiness is to undermine the current image of fasting, and no doubt to remove from it, in some people's eyes, part of its attractions. For most men, indeed, "fasting" evokes suffering. Fasting seems like one of the most costly sacrifices, demanding a heroic generosity. Therefore, an easy fast seems suspect, defective. What use is it to fast, if not to make oneself suffer?

This way of seeing fasting is not only general today, but it has deep historical roots in the Judeo-Christian tradition in particular. In surveying the Bible and the literature of ancient monasticism, we often met it. Therefore, there is no question of removing it as unsatisfactory or erroneous. All I can say is that it does not correspond to my own experience. Wrongly or rightly I set myself to fasting so gently and gradually that I do not remember ever having made a violent effort. In the course of the years, the regular fast has entered into my life almost imperceptibly, becoming a happy and beloved habit without my having to suffer from it. Sometimes, of course, I have had to begin the day feeling rather low, have had to resist feelings of hunger, and use a little patience. But on the whole, the dominant impression has not been that of a painful tension. On the contrary, I have lived the discovery of the fast as a joyful liberation.

What I have just said about the years when I was learning to fast is still more true of the following years. The regular fast, becoming a weekday exercise all year, is for me less an effort than a very agreeable way of life. I practice it with pleasure, so appreciating its advantages that I regret its interruptions.

This probably would be the opinion of the majority in a community that would adopt it. In this domain, as in others, habit is the chief factor, and therefore, let it be said in passing, I am today persuaded that the accounts of the prolonged fasts which abound in ancient monastic literature, have every chance of being historically true. To this common effect of habit, which facilitates everything, is added the singular well-being procured by the daily fast at the blessed hour when it comes to an end and makes its purifying effects felt with more vigor. But does not making the fast thus habitual, easy and even pleasant, devaluate and even denature it?

The question is crucial, for it touches the very essence of the regular fast. By nature, the latter is not an exceptional act, a transient sacrifice, but a custom and a way of life. This regularity removes from it the heroic character that seems to establish the value of the act of fasting. What is more, it contradicts the medical definition of the fast as a halt in the normal rhythm of meals.

To these objections I reply without hesitation that the fast, by becoming regular, in no way loses its beneficial effects, either spiritual or physiological. Of course, it no longer demands the momentary expenditure of energy that seems to give it merit, but every day it sets a man to fasting, that is, it places him in a state of digestive inactivity and of interior liberty, where he feels more himself and close to God. This sort of daily retreat continues to pacify his body and soul. Perhaps even the depth of the peace it procures is, in large measure, the result of its dailyness.

However paradoxical this may appear, I believe in the value of a regular observance which one can make one's own without great effort and practice without much trouble, indeed with a true pleasure, felt by one's whole being. Is this an effect of my age or my cowardice? While I respect and admire those who live the fast differently, I envisage it for myself as a happy way of life, to which one can approach in small steps, and which fashions a man little by little. There is no need to strain towards it or think much about it. When one has introduced it into one's life, it is enough to let it act.

As with the individual, so the community that would embrace the regular fast, would no doubt be deeply and imperceptibly transformed by it. The monks would soon cease considering it as a distressing penance. What happened to me might even happen to them, that finding the practice of fasting so sweet and beneficial, they would go beyond St. Benedict's horarium and calendar and take the one meal a day, as their perpetual norm. Thus one avoids the jerkiness of a varied and intermittent practice, which risks paradoxically being much more laborious.

Still, I do not wish to overlook certain merits of the supple regime prescribed by the Rule. With its remissions and variations, it does better in avoiding routine, and while remaining "regular," it obliges to renewed efforts. In that way it corresponds better to the medical definition cited above (Chapter II, n. 47–51) and to the sacrificial images evoked currently by the word. Fasting in that way would relate the monks closer to the occasional fasters, that is, practically all those who practice fasting today for different reasons and in diverse forms.

Minor advantages of fasting

But in calculating in this way what some monastic communities interested in fasting might do, I seem to be launching out into a pure utopia. Where indeed is anyone seriously thinking about such a thing? For that, fasting would first have "to be loved" with a powerful love.

Thus we are brought back again to the search for motives capable of stirring us to make this experiment. I believe I have stated the principal ones, by enumerating some of the meanings of fasting. For monks, it is less a question of external reasons, such as protests, witness or solidarity with the Third World, than of an improvement of human and spiritual well-being produced by the very act of fasting. But to this fundamental benefit, which by itself would amply justify the whole enterprise, can be added subsidiary considerations, which are not to be despised.

The first of these secondary advantages is the time saved. Sitting down to eat once instead of three times a day is to eliminate from the schedule two gatherings that can be replaced with other actions. To tell the truth, the net gain is not so easy to calculate because of the prolongation of the one meal. He who eats only once in twenty-four hours necessarily spends more time at table than at one of the three usual meals. As I have said, my daily dinner takes me a full hour. While taking into account a certain slowness proper to a solitary who reads while eating, it remains true that cenobites themselves would probably be obliged to remain at table much longer than they do now, even at their chief meal. This duration, while perhaps not equalling the sum total of the three present meals, would not be much different.

But the time saved by fasting is still considerable. Think of all that goes with the meals: the preparation of the food and of the table, serving the dishes and removing them, the washing and putting things away, not to speak of the comings and goings, the gathering of the community, the prayers before meals and grace afterwards. By doing all that only once a day, one gets rid of a heavy material burden and the spirit feels more free.

A second benefit of the fast would be to restore to the monastic meal a consistency and deportment that it tends to lose at the present time. Even from its beginning, breakfast has been taken furtively, so to speak, despite the increasing quantity of food eaten. But recently supper also often has the same furtive and neglected aspect: arrival and departure at will, self-service, no common prayer or reading. Evidently the influence of the world does not explain everything. If that influence is strong in so many monasteries, it is because it has found fertile ground there. The weight of the ceremonial meal seems excessive when it is felt more than once a day.

This inconvenience would disappear with fasting. No one would be tempted to cheapen the one and only meal. This meal would gain in both natural and religious dignity, while the mere running in and out of the refectory, unworthy of a community of men of God, would disappear.

Finally, fasting would introduce into the monastic horarium a suppleness and flexibility lacking to it. The monotony of three meals, eaten every day of the year at about the same time, would give way to changes that would set in relief the different seasons and days. This differentiation is also important for one like me, who dispenses with fasting only on Sundays and feast days, but it would be still more so if one followed the dispositions of the Rule. The result would be not only a variety favorable to human equilibrium, but also, in possible connection with a renewed Eucharistic practice, an emphasis on the Lord's Day as a meeting with the risen Christ and the awaiting of his return.[17]

Outline of a method

Since I have descended to the practical level, perhaps some concrete suggestions on attaining the regular fast are expected of me. In this domain more than in any other, only personal experience counts, and mine is limited. However,

17. Suggested by my article "Eucharistie et vie monastique," in *Collectanea Cisterciensia* 48 (1986), p. 120–130. English translation in *Worship* 59 (1985), p. 498–510.

I shall tell what it has taught me, in the hope that these modest observations will be helpful.

First of all, I suggest starting slowly, reducing one of the superfluous meals little by little, then the other. These gradual reductions are normally accompanied by increasing the meal to be retained: fasting is not starvation. At the end of the process one will be eating less, of course, but it is not necessary or opportune to impose this diminution of quantity on oneself from the beginning. It will result naturally from the fact that one eats only once a day.

I say the same in regard to the diversity of foods and number of dishes. In this matter one can begin by transferring elsewhere what one suppresses from the "useless" meal. Simplifications will come later. The important thing is to advance step by step, without great forward leaps or retreats to the rear, taking the time to get used to the changes.

This absence of haste should be accompanied by a true liberty. We should not feel obliged to attain a definite result, but go along tranquilly in the discovery of what can be done. We should know how to let up on the reins, as riders say, to yield for a moment to the horse straining at its bit, then tightening up on the rein again quietly when the animal has had its satisfaction. Therefore if we feel worn out one day, we should grant ourselves a relaxation without anxiety or a bad conscience, knowing that the will remains and will resume its journey.

To be free and without care makes a person strong. The conquest of fasting should develop in a joyous peace, and nothing favors this peace so much as giving oneself up to the will of God, by always remaining ready to bend to circumstances, to "necessity," as St. Francis said.[18]

What I have said about circumspection in the reduction of the quantity and diversity of food, which are not to be reduced too soon, derives from a more general axiom of great importance: to set forth the questions in the right order. Fasting is one thing, abstinence another. Certainly these two renunciations can be mingled, one reinforcing the other, thus attacking simultaneously along the whole front. But such bravery is not my style, nor is it to be recommended to most.

Let us recall Rancé and his first Trappists. Because they threw themselves into the regular fast with a diet heavily loaded with privations, they experienced a failure whose consequences were long and regrettable. Their example suggests that fasting and abstinence should not be combined too quickly. If we wish to arrive at a stable practice of fasting, it is important not only to work towards it progressively, something that Rancé and his disciples did not do, but also to confront it with a sufficient diet.

Thus it seems wise to recall constantly that if fasting is often accompanied by abstinence and rationing in the documents on the subject, still it is not intrinsically connected

18. Francis of Assisi, *Regula* I, 9, 13; II, 3, 9.

with these retrenchments. Fasting is merely to await the hour of the meal with an empty stomach, without this meal being in itself subject to particular limitations. The only limitation mentioned by St. Benedict is abstinence from meat, and I can testify that it causes no difficulty for the horarium of the Rule. I would fear that the stricter abstinence of the Carthusians and Cistercians, of which I have no experience, might be an obstacle to the regular fast, at least in the delicate period when one is beginning and getting used to it.

Whether the fast is considered in itself or together with rationing and abstinence all food discipline in the monastic setting aims at becoming a permanent discipline. The aim is to enter an enduring, even a definitive state, rather than imposing temporary restrictions, followed by relaxations. Modest progress that can be maintained is preferable to ambitious acts that cannot be continued. Instead of removing violently and temporarily something necessary, we shall aim at getting a better grip on what is "necessary," separating it from what seems necessary but is not truly so.

This peaceful work of research and reduction can orient our efforts during Lent. Usually Lent is conceived as a time of exceptional generosity, in violent contrast not only with the Paschal season but also with the whole year. For the monk whose whole life should resemble Lent, as St. Benedict says, it is natural that the contrast be much less.[19]

19. RB 49:1. Cf. Cassian, *Conferences* 21, 29–30.

Instead of the monk's doing in Lent what he does not do at other times, he can use this period of grace and effort as an experimental field to set in order the regime he will practice all year. Simplifying his diet and reducing it to real need is no doubt much less exalting a task than imposing harsh privations on oneself temporarily, but if this simplification continues, is not the profit from it much better?

Beyond the issue of Lent, the issue here is a whole way of conceiving mortification and sacrifice. Not long ago, in line with St. Thérèse of the Child Jesus, we were taught that the best kind of mortification was that of many little sacrifices that keep the soul in practice, without giving it cause for pride in itself. This sort of guerrilla warfare, for which I have the highest respect, was not an invention of the Saint of Lisieux. It is perfectly described in one of the Fathers' apophthegmata.[20] But however profitable it may be, it does not lead to the end we have in view. It can even turn us away from it by impeding our quest for any result of a certain amplitude, demanding a long effort.

To attain the regular fast, something other than this harassment of small mortifications is needed. What is at stake is a complete and methodical transformation of a way of life. Without scattering its attention on a multitude of details, the mind must arm itself with a deep and tranquil resolution. When meal time comes, it should restrain itself

20. Apophthegm N592I–2, in L. Régnault, pp. 215–217 (no. 1592/1–2).

from generous impulses and take without misgiving everything it has decided to take. Henceforth, mortification consists in an overall plan of reform, rather than in a multitude of small vexations, which, at least in certain natures, run the risk of arousing anxiety or turning into masochism.

I shall end this series of practical suggestions by noting a surprising phenomenon that we should be able to profit by: the lessening of hunger as the day advances. Often a person will begin the day poorly, with very little vigor, and will wonder if he will last until evening. But quite unexpectedly, his strength does not continue to wane, but on the contrary increases until meal time. His general tone of being is quite low at the beginning of the morning, but rises with the sun. At noon it is at its zenith, and instead of declining with the day, it stays at the same height: the afternoon hours, when the fast exerts its full effect, are when he feels at his best. Resist, therefore, the pangs of hunger that sometimes strike at the beginning of the day! The resistance and waiting will be rewarded. If one's spirits are too low, a glass of water will fool the hunger without seriously damaging the fast.

It will be noted that everything I have just written is addressed to the individual seeking to practice the regular fast, without taking into account the social framework in which this search takes place. For a solitary like me, this framework scarcely exists. How can a monk living in community make such suggestions his own? That problem I leave undiscussed. Clearly many difficulties are to be foreseen.

One of the chief difficulties, however, is tending to disappear these days. I pointed out earlier that in a number of monasteries, supper is often an informal meal, analogous to breakfast. This degradation, though debatable in itself, at least has the advantage of leaving more liberty. Instead of a community exercise at which one must be present, the buffet supper is only an optional gathering at which absence is not noticed.

Supper, thus assimilated to breakfast, remains nonetheless a more respectable entity from the historical point of view. In principle, we should not start the effort of simplification with supper, but with this latest newcomer and foreign import, namely breakfast. This has never had a communitarian character that prevents its being dispensed with.

However, in this domain considerations of principle are of little importance. The obstacles to be surmounted in the midst of community life are too many for one not to use the maximum of realism and of suppleness, paying attention to circumstances and profiting by every opportunity.

Two inconveniences resulting from one meal a day

Before leaving this plane of practical considerations we must listen to a reproach sometimes levelled at the regular fast: that of making the one meal too important. Physiologically, some people cannot take such a quantity of food at one time. From an ascetical point of view good authors long ago have warned against the desire to eat too much at one time: it is better to take less and take it more often.[21]

Under its medical aspect, this criticism reminds us that the regular fast assumes normal health. If a person has a delicate stomach, there is no question of exposing such a one to gastritis or an ulcer by fasting. But this consideration of the sick should not turn the healthy away from fasting. In fact, the rather copious meal that the one dinner necessarily is, is borne without difficulty. It would certainly be an abuse to erect into a medical law the division of the daily quantity of food into three or even more meals.

Moreover it is good to remember that medical theories are not immutable. I hear it said that the medical schools were recently inclined to multiply small meals but now they incline towards making them fewer and more substantial. On this point as on every other, a certain relativism should keep us from following too quickly and too confidently the advice of "science." Monastic life has its laws that cannot always bend to these changing pieces of advice. While remaining attentive to the contemporary science of nutrition, we have chiefly to listen to a voice that comes from a greater distance. When we have a long tradition behind us, the wisest thing to do when today's medicine disapproves of us, is to wait until tomorrow's medicine approves us.

---

21. Thus an Irish rule of the ninth century (*Rule of Tallaght* 44), cited by E. de Bhaldraithe, "Monasticism in the United States," p. 8. See note 7 above.

From the ascetic point of view, it is true that someone like Cassian blames those who prefer to wait longer in order to gorge themselves at one sitting. It is better, he says, to eat more often, and each time to remain a little hungry.[22] But it does not follow that the principle of one daily meal has been disavowed. On the contrary, it was to establish it that he counselled against meals at longer intervals. What Cassian disapproves of is waiting two or more days in order to have the satisfaction of filling one's belly. According to him, the right measure is to eat daily, but not more than two small loaves of bread.

It is wrong therefore to invoke the doctrine of the Fathers to condemn the regular fast. The only important conclusion to draw is that the one daily meal should be sober, indeed a little less than filling. What Cassian said of the two small loaves of bread in the Egyptian desert is also valid for the three dishes of the Benedictine Rule: it is good for the monk, when rising from the table, to still feel unsatisfied.

The place of fasting in Christianity

Besides these concrete difficulties proposed against fasting, modern Christianity probably needs to be freed from one great objection, either conscious or latent, which might turn it away from fasting. At first sight the New Testament

22. *Conferences* 2, 24, which probably inspired the *Rule of Tallaght*, which should be interpreted in the same way.

scarcely recommends it. The Gospels speak of it chiefly to criticize the way in which the Pharisees practice it,[23] and to excuse Christ's disciples for not practicing it.[24] The letters of St. Paul frequently assert the Christian's liberty in regard to the dietary rules that others claim to impose on him.[25] All that seems to display quite a detached attitude towards fasting and other similar practices. Is it really worthwhile after Christ to attach such importance to it?

I shall not repeat the New Testament texts cited in the historical review of fasting. These testimonies, starting with Anna the prophetess and including the Apostle of the Gentiles, and Jesus himself, show the vitality of fasting in the Jewish world in which the Church was born, and its transmission to the Church as a natural element of the Christian life. If Jesus dispensed his disciples from fasting while he was with them, he said they would return to it when he left. If Paul vindicated Christian liberty against all forced abstinence, he spoke with pride of the fasts he frequently accomplished in Christ's service[26] and of the "harsh blows" he inflicted on his body "to reduce it to servitude."[27]

---

23. Mt 6:16; Lk 18:12.
24. Mt 9:14–17 and parallels. Cf. Mt 11:19; Lk 7:34.
25. Rm 14:1–23 (cf. Ga 4:10); 1 Co 8–10; Col 2:16–23; 1 Tm 4:3–5.
26. See 2 Co 6:5 ("watchings and fasts") and 11:27. The "frequent fasts" of this last passage seems distinguished from the mere "hunger and thirst" (cf. 1 Co 4:11) undergone involuntarily.
27. 1 Co 9:27, universally understood by the Fathers as meaning fasting.

Furthermore, it is hard to see how such a discipline could be missing from a religious tradition that which begins with the story of a sin connected with eating and ends with the hope of a never-ending banquet.[28] In between there are Christ and his forty days without eating or drinking, the gift of his body and blood signified by the bread and the wine from which the Christian receives his daily nourishment. In such a real and symbolic framework it would be strange if eating and fasting were negligible values. If they have become such, is it not the result of a deadly distraction from which we should escape as soon as possible?

To love fasting

St. Benedict's axiom remains the golden rule. "To love fasting" sums it up. In the list of maxims of which it is part, only one other virtue is proposed to the monk with the same verb *amare*, namely, chastity. "To love fasting.... To love chastity." The analogy of these two patterns of behavior is obvious and justifies bringing them together. For a monk, to be chaste is to renounce carnal union completely; to fast is to renounce nourishment for a while. Both abstinences are worthy of being loved, the first because of the high possibilities it offers for union with God, the second for the help it affords in attaining the same. The monk loves chastity because it frees

28. Cf. J.-D. Nordmann, "Le jeûne aujourd'hui," in *Sources* 9 (1983), p. 58–71 (see p. 60).

him to love more. He loves fasting because it purifies the body and pacifies the soul, giving joy and freedom to the whole being.

Trial and effort are not lacking to those who wish to remain chaste. Long effort is also necessary to attain the fast and to maintain it. But in each case the attraction of a superior good is accompanied by the daily experience of its benefits. It is this satisfaction found in fasting that has led me to write, and it is what I predict and wish for whoever wants to try it.

APPENDIX

Two horariums of the Regular Fast

The Rule of the Master and that of St. Benedict were written in Italy one after the other in the first-two thirds of the sixth century. We give a summary of the first and a translation of the second.

Days of fast and time of repast[1]

The community eats its meal at the sixth hour (midday) on Thursdays and Sundays and at the ninth hour (3 P.M.) the other days.[2] In Lent, the meal is pushed back until after Vespers, a time that also holds for the Wednesdays, Fridays and Saturdays during the two weeks preceding Lent.

The sick eat three hours earlier, that is, at the third hour (9 A.M.) or at the sixth hour, when the brothers eat at the sixth or ninth hour. Children less than twelve years old fast

1. *The Rule of the Master*, Cistercian Studies no. 6 (Kalamazoo, MI: Cistercian Publications, 1977), pp. 187–190 (RM 28). See also p. 204: the eight days preceding Christmas are assimilated to Lent, and the season of Christmas to Epiphany is assimilated to Paschal time (RM 45, 2–7).
2. On these two days there is a second meal in the evening in the summer, but not in winter (RM 27, 28).

in winter only on Wednesdays, Fridays and Saturdays, eating their meal at the sixth hour the other days. In summer they eat at noon on Wednesdays, Fridays and Saturdays, at the third hour the other days.

Brothers on a journey do not fast in summer. In winter they fast until evening Wednesdays, Fridays and Saturdays; the other days they eat twice, at noon and in the evening.

In Paschal time the community meal is eaten at noon. On Thursdays and Sundays there is also a supper in the evening.[3] On the other days, the advancement of the one meal to noon suffices to show that the monks are not fasting.

The times for the brothers' meals[4]

From holy Easter to Pentecost the brothers eat at noon and take supper in the evening. Beginning with Pentecost and continuing throughout the summer, the monks fast until mid-afternoon on Wednesdays and Fridays, unless they are working in the fields or the summer heat is oppressive.

On the other days they eat dinner at noon. Indeed, the abbot may decide that they should continue to eat dinner at noon every day if they have work in the fields or if the summer heat remains extreme. Similarly, he should so regulate and arrange all matters that souls may be saved and

3. The monks also eat supper every day during the octave of Easter (RM 27, 34).
4. Timothy Fry, O.S.B., ed., *RB 1980: The Rule of Saint Benedict in English* (Collegeville, MN: The Liturgical Press, 1981), Chapter 41.

the brothers may go about their activities without justifiable grumbling.

From the thirteenth of September to the beginning of Lent, they always take their meal in mid-afternoon. Finally, from the beginning of Lent to Easter, they eat towards evening. Let Vespers be celebrated early enough so that there is no need for a lamp while eating, and that everything can be finished by daylight. Indeed, at all times let supper or the hour of the fast-day meal be so scheduled that everything can be done by daylight.

Designed by Fiona Cecile Clarke, the CLUNY MEDIA *logo*
depicts a monk at work in the scriptorium,
with a cat sitting at his feet.

The monk represents our mission to emulate
the invaluable contributions of the monks
of Cluny in preserving the libraries of the West,
our strivings to know and love the truth.

The cat at the monk's feet is Pangur Bán, from the
eponymous Irish poem of the 9th century.
The anonymous poet compares his scholarly
pursuit of truth with the cat's happy hunting of mice.
The depiction of Pangur Bán is an homage to the work
of the monks of Irish monasteries and a sign
of the joy we at Cluny take in our trade.

"Messe ocus Pangur Bán,
cechtar nathar fria saindan:
bíth a menmasam fri seilgg,
mu memna céin im saincheirdd."

Made in the USA
Monee, IL
13 September 2026

62981949R00111